Inside an Emotional Health Program

A Field Study of Workplace Assistance for Troubled Employees

William J. Sonnenstuhl

ILR Press
New York State School of
Industrial and Labor Relations
Cornell University

Cover design: Kathleen Dalton

Library of Congress Number: 86-7145
ISBN: 0-87546-119-0 (cloth)
       0-87546-120-4 (paper)

Library of Congress Cataloging in Publication Data
Sonnenstuhl, William J., 1946–
     Inside an emotional health program.

     Bibliography: p.
     Includes index.
     1. Mental health services. 2. Occupational health
services. 3. Industrial psychiatry. I. Title.
[DNLM: 1. Mental Health Services. 2. Occupational
Health Services. WA 495 S699i]
RC969.P8S66   1986   362.2'0425   86-7145
ISBN 0-87546-119-0
ISBN 0-87546-120-4 (pbk.)

Copies may be ordered from
ILR Press
New York State School of
Industrial and Labor Relations
Cornell University
Ithaca, New York 14851-0952

Printed by Braun-Brumfield in the United States of America
5   4   3   2   1

Dedicated to
Mr. R. Brinkley Smithers and
the Christopher D. Smithers Foundation,
for support and encouragement

Contents

Preface

I have worked both as a consultant to, and as an administrator of, corporate emotional health programs. This study grew out of those experiences and my curiosity about how employees actually decide to use such programs. In conducting this research project, I have attempted to bracket those experiences by using a social constructionist perspective on the study of trouble and by allowing the employees and members of the emotional health staff to tell their own program experiences in their own words. Such an approach inevitably highlights the differences in actors' perspectives, and this helped me to understand the social complexity of emotional health programs in a way that I could never have if I had relied upon my insider's knowledge and experience only.

A number of people gave me invaluable advice and assistance in conducting this field study and in preparing the manuscript. I should like particularly to acknowledge the generous support that I received from Edwin Schur, Eliot Freidson, and Wolf Heydebrand, who were my teachers at New York University and whose understanding of social control and deviance, occupations, and organizational theory helped me to understand emotional health programs anew. I am also particularly appreciative of Harrison Trice's encouragement and generosity. From the project's inception to its publication, he freely shared with me his fieldwork experiences and the fruits of his research on industrial alcoholism and employee assistance programs. I also appreciate the comments and encouragement that I received from Peter Conrad, Richard Maisel, Caroline Persell, Paul Roman, Alan Sadovnich, and Joseph Schneider. And, I am appreciative of my editors—particularly Janet Wagner, whose probing questions prodded me to clarify my written thoughts.

I also should like to thank *Contemporary Drug Problems* for their permission to reprint sections of chapter 4, which originally appeared as "Understanding EAP Self-Referral: Towards a Social Network Approach."

1. The evolution of emotional health programs

The corporate emotional health program (EHP) is a relatively new phenomenon in the workplace. An outgrowth of alcoholism programs of World War II, emotional health programs began to proliferate in the early 1970s, when the focus of the programs began to shift from alcoholism to any personal problem that affects job performance.

Companies use a variety of names for their programs: counseling, employee assistance, troubled employee, mental wellness, special health services, and alcoholism (Weiss 1980). Some are located within a company's personnel department and others within a company's medical department; some are administered by alcoholism specialists and others by mental health specialists (e.g., psychiatrists, psychologists, social workers); some offer employees extensive in-house treatment services, and others refer employees to community treatment services.

Regardless of their title or structure, all are concerned with preventing, identifying, and treating personal problems that adversely affect job performance. For the purpose of this book, an emotional health program is any program operating within a work organization for the purpose of identifying troubled employees and delivering mental health services (e.g., psychotherapy, behavior modification, alcoholism counseling) to them. Services are provided either within the corporation, within the community, or within a combination of the two. This definition assumes that the program is administered and staffed by people who are knowledgeable about such therapies and capable of referring employees to therapists (e.g., psychiatrists, psychologists, social workers, and alcoholism counselors) in the community.

As the number of corporate programs has grown, the mass media have focused increasing attention on them. A *New York Times* advertisement proclaimed, "EAP [employee assistance program]: Helping your employees builds a healthier business," and in *Savvy* magazine journalist Patricia O'Toole (1980) blasted "the menace of the corporate shrink." O'Toole, contending that emotional health programs undermine empolyees' civil liberties, stated that she cannot understand why people use them for help with their personal problems.

> Corporate psychological counseling is dangerous not by design but by nature. Few corporations are malevolent, the vast majority are scrupulous, and employees seeking help don't have a thought of surrendering an inch of personal freedom. But despite the good intentions in all quarters, the move to bring the intricacies of psychological assistance inside the corporation has laid the groundwork for the day when employers could own their employees body and soul. (1980, 52)

She concluded that workers refer themselves to such programs because they irrationally fear freedom and wish to escape from it into the protective arms of paternalism.

O'Toole raises some provocative questions. Indeed, if emotional health programs act as sophisticated social control agencies and undermine civil liberties, why do employees refer themselves to them for help? Unfortunately, O'Toole's conclusion that employees use such programs because they irrationally fear freedom and wish to escape from it into corporate paternalism tells us little about how employees actually choose to use an emotional health program or what the consequences of program use are, issues that are central to the case study of "Corpco" later in these pages.

Nevertheless, O'Toole's view of emotional health programs

as agencies of social control is an important perception, for, in a sense, the evolution of these programs may be seen as a process of refining employer influence over employee behavior. Social control in work organizations is a practical necessity. Every organization—government agency, business, or social service—must satisfy some basic goals if it is to survive. For example, companies must procure raw materials from the environment, convert those raw materials into some product, and introduce the product into the marketplace for consumption. This means delegating responsibility to individuals and evaluating how well the responsible individuals perform. Traditionally, business managers have maintained that it is their prerogative to delegate such responsibilities and to dictate the terms of performance evaluation, and they have been very reluctant to share these decisions with workers. Hence ideological conflict: managers and workers argue over how work is to be structured, how job performance standards are to be created, and how work is to be evaluated (e.g., Edwards 1979). The conflict's uneasy resolution can be seen in such experiments as the "Z" organization (Ouchi and Jaeger 1978) and quality of working life demonstrations (O'Toole 1973) and in such movements as self-management (Vanek 1975) and workplace democracy (Whyte et al. 1983; Zwerdling 1980). The resolution, however, generally allows management to plan its business activities so that the organization has the best chances of survival.

In order to ensure that employees and work groups carry out its plans, management has introduced a wide variety of control systems into organizations, among which are budgets; performance appraisals; computerized management information systems; books of rules, practices, and procedures; and production reports (Lawler 1976). All are designed to give management feedback on how well its goals are being met.

The most effective form of social control, however, comes from employing workers who accept management's norms, beliefs, and morals and can be expected to act accordingly. When such employees deviate from management's expectations, they, in effect, discipline themselves and correct their own performance. Consequently when hiring, organizations try to select those with the "right" beliefs, and in order to ensure that workers retain the right beliefs, organizations conduct training and education programs.

Discipline is the principal form of social control used in the workplace to ensure conformance with job standards, and since the 1880s, the sanctions used to discipline employees have become less punitive and more therapeutic. In part, this change reflects different philosophies adopted by management to mediate their historical conflicts with workers, and in part, it reflects legal and social constraints on their ability to fire employees.

Early philosophies of personnel relations

Between 1880 and 1936, labor-management relations were often marked by violence (e.g., Brandes 1970; Boyer and Morais 1970). Incipient unions struggled to organize workers for better pay and living conditions; managers struck back with private armies often composed of Pinkerton agents and local thugs. Bloodshed ensued, and by the turn of the century, there was a severe crisis. In order to mitigate this violent relationship, managers adopted a succession of philosophies: social Darwinism, scientific management, social welfarism, and human relations.

Social Darwinism (Carneiro 1967; Peel 1972) emerged during the latter part of the nineteenth century, when large numbers of immigrants entered the American labor force. Predominantly Catholics from southern and eastern European countries, they threatened by their sheer numbers to overwhelm the culture of native-born Protestants. By asserting Darwin's concept of survival of the fittest, social Darwinism emphasized the moral superiority of the dominant Protestant group. Reflected in the workplace, where managers were generally Protestants and workers were Catholic immigrants, social Darwinism argued that superior performance emerged from natural, impersonal, competitive processes that should be allowed to operate freely (Trice and Beyer 1984a, Perrow 1972). Managers were intolerant of poor performers and fired them. They ruthlessly pitted workers against one another and admonished them to work hard, to compete to the best of their ability, and to accept defeat as an expression of inevitable evolutionary processes. Managers characterized themselves as biologically superior individuals and unproductive workers as biologically unfit.

During the mid-1880s, the New Thought Movement modified social Darwinism's harsh biological determinism with a somewhat more optimistic explanation of managers' success and workers' failure (Perrow 1972). This movement held that positive thinking is the key to business success. Managers characterized themselves as being morally superior and possessing an abundance of will power, perceived cooperative workers as having "proper thoughts," and described unproductive workers as unwilling to try. This explanation was attractive to those workers who could not accept their failure as biologically determined. While this theory held out some hope to those workers who were willing to try harder, it did little to improve labor and management relations.

Scientific management or Taylorism (Taylor 1911) also emerged during the 1890s and had a great affinity with social Darwinism. It sought to make the harsh policies of Darwinism fairer by couching its ideology in science and instructing workers in how to be more competitive.

Taylorism assumed that the most rational way to organize the workplace is for management to appropriate the knowledge of the craftsperson, arrange the knowledge into discrete tasks, and give the discrete tasks to workers to perform. Taylorism held that workers are motivated by money—the more discrete the tasks, the easier the work, the more productivity, and the more money for labor and management. The cause of unsatisfactory performance is either poorly defined tasks or "bad" employees. If poorly defined tasks and rewards cause unsatisfactory performance, management should undertake a scientific study to redefine them more appropriately. If the problem is caused by a bad employee, he or she is fired. Although workers have always fought against Taylorism, it underlies modern management theory (Drucker 1974). Indeed, Harry Braverman (1974) contends that it is being applied increasingly to office workers, whether they are clericals, professionals, or middle managers. In reality, very few full-scale scientific management studies have ever been undertaken because of the great cost involved. According to David Noble (1977), Taylorism is not a scientific theory or a method of organization, but an ideological justification for management's continued domination in the workplace.

During the same period that Taylorism emerged, industrial welfare work evolved (Brandes 1970; Carter 1977; Edwards 1979; Eilbert 1959; Nelson and Campbell 1972). Social welfarism or industrial betterment, which grew out of the activities of a few paternalistic employers and humanitarian reformers, was established in Europe during the 1850s and in American industry during the 1880s. After the passage of the Sherman Anti-Trust Act in 1890, corporations became more welfare-oriented because betterment programs gave them the image, at least, of being socially responsible (Brandes 1970).

The goals of social welfarism were to create a "new corporate man" and thus forestall union organizing. Unlike Taylorism, industrial welfare work had no definite set of practices, but its underlying assumption appears to have been that employees are motivated by job security and by good working conditions and that, provided these, workers will perform as expected. The National Civic Federation, a prominent supporter of social welfarism policies in the early 1900s, defined industrial welfare work as

> involv[ing] special consideration for physical comfort wherever labor is performed, opportunities for recreation, educational advantages, and the providing of suitable sanitary homes ... plans for saving and lending

money, and provisions for insurance and pensions. (quoted in Nelson and Campbell 1972, 3)

Welfare programs usually provided for some form of employee representation in a company-sponsored union (Brandes 1970). These unions were not independent and therefore unable to truly bargain with management.

Employers supporting social welfarism stressed their philanthropic motives but also their desire to secure a stable labor force, "decrease the floating element," promote harmonious relations and worker loyalty, combat unionism, and ensure against strikes (Carter 1977; Nelson and Campbell 1972). John Patterson, president of National Cash Register and an enthusiastic supporter of industrial welfare work, adopted the slogan It Pays and maintained that he could calculate the profits on his welfare expenditures. Frederick Taylor, commenting on a strike at National Cash Register, stated that Patterson had it backwards and that "semi-philanthropic schemes should follow rather than preceding the solution of wage questions."

In general, Taylorism and welfare work were introduced into different kinds of work sites. Taylorism was adopted by the machine industry, which was located in urban areas. Welfare work was adopted by department stores, textile mills, and mines, places that either were isolated or employed a large number of women. Because of their philosophical differences, Taylorism and welfare work were not usually introduced into the same workplaces.

Eventually, however, welfare programs came to be viewed by management as just another economic reward given to those employees who complied. Typifying attitudes at such diverse industries as General Electric, United States Steel, and Pullman, Patrick McCormick's letter of 1919 to the employees of International Harvester captures the sentiment perfectly: "As you know, our Pension Plan is a purely voluntary expression of the company's desire to stand by the men who have stood by it" (quoted in Edwards 1979, 93). Partially as a consequence of this change in perspective, by 1920 scientific management and welfarism combined to form the new field of personnel administration (Eilbert 1959; Ritzer and Trice 1969).

During the late twenties, the growth in welfare programs slackened, and many companies dropped them. Generally, they retained the more practical ones, such as medical care and pension plans, and dropped the educational, recreational, and religious elements. The number of employee representation programs, however, continued to grow because companies saw them as an inexpensive and effective means of minimizing union threats.

By the thirties, labor and management relations had turned violent once again, and the federal govenment, forced to intercede, passed the National Labor Relations Act. The act outlawed employee representation programs, declaring that it was an unfair labor practice for business to support a company union or to use hiring and firing to encourage membership in one. This so actively encouraged the growth of unions that by 1943 union membership was triple that of 1935 (Brandes 1970). Since the struggle against unions was lost, there was little reason to continue supporting social welfarism.

Human relations theory was developed in the 1930s, but its roots go back to the mental hygiene movement of the early part of the twentieth century, which espoused the beliefs and values of the Protestant ethic (Davis 1938). It stressed that individuals could get ahead if they took responsibility for their own lives, worked hard, were thrifty, pursued practical ends with the best available means, and behaved rationally, not letting their emotions get in the way of progress. People who could not take responsibility for their own lives could learn to do so with the help of mental hygienists.

These ideas also formed the basis of the human relations school. Human relations theory emphasized that workers were tractable and wanted to be led, that they wanted to feel united in some cause bigger than themselves, and that their irrational feelings prevented them from cooperating with management. According to this theory, unless workers and management

8

cooperate, everyone fails. Management fosters cooperation by paying attention to workers' irrational sentiments, discovering common purposes, and making a purposeful effort to structure a cooperative organization. Counseling programs are one method of managing employees' irrationality.

The human relations school traced its origins to the work of Elton Mayo, who believed that poor work performance was caused by workers' irrational thoughts. To combat this irrationality, he recommended that companies develop psychiatric clinics "to eliminate eccentricities from the 'normal' persons engaged in industry" (Mayo 1923, 483). For example, he claimed that workers' demands for increased wages or improved working conditions are often the symptoms of "maladjustment or distortion" in "average normal" people. When they are untreated, these minor irrationalities accumulate, causing eventually a breakdown in the company. The clinic, then, by treating the irrational thoughts of "normal" workers prevented a breakdown in either the individual employee or the organization. During the 1920s, R. H. Macy and Company (Anderson 1944) and the Metropolitan Life Insurance Company (Giberson 1936) developed full-time psychiatric clinics, but it was not until after publication of the Hawthorne studies that Mayo's ideas became widely accepted.

The Hawthorne studies were conducted at Western Electric during the 1920s and 1930s and reported by Fritz Roethlisberger and William Dickson in their classic *Management and the Worker* (1939). These studies were interpreted as dramatic proof that workers behaved irrationally and that management could control that irrationality by adopting counseling programs and developing a cooperative attitude toward employees. Originally, these studies were undertaken to examine the relationship between lighting conditions and productivity. To the great surprise of the researchers, the productivity of both the experimental group, whose lighting was varied, and that of the control group, whose lighting was unchanged, increased during the experiment. After manipulating other working conditions (e.g., temperature, method of payment, rest periods, work rules) and finding that no matter how the conditions changed, both the experimental and control goups increased their productivity, the researchers hypothesized that the increased production of the workers was caused by the very fact that they were being studied. This phenomenon was called the "Hawthorne effect." The researchers further reasoned that productivity was increased because throughout the experiments workers were asked for their opinions and comments about the tests and the increased attention raised the workers' morale. They hypothesized that the heightened morale increased productivity.

In order to further test their hypothesis, the researchers began to interview plant employees to find out what was on their minds, and W. Lloyd Warner undertook a field study in the plant. They discovered that workers, when uninvolved in the experiments, restricted output and penalized those who produced more than the group had informally agreed to produce and that some supervisors were rated as better leaders than others because they treated employees decently. Returning to their laboratory observations, the researchers set up an experiment that confirmed that workers restricted output; established a fair day's rate; subjected "rate busters" to ostracism, sabotage, and physical threats; and falsified records. The researchers labeled such behavior irrational and stressed the lack of cooperation with rational management and the lack of identification with the rational goals of the company. The workers' explanations of their behavior (e.g., fear of producing too much, which could mean that some would be laid off) were dismissed as mere rationalizations.

The Hawthorne findings led to a general theory of industrial relations that recognized that factory life has a complex internal social organization of cliques and status hierarchies. Roethlisberger and Dickson concluded that the work groups, not management, regulated productivity by defining performance standards and by using group pressure to prevent rate busting.

One strategy used by management to regain control of the

production process was the development of a personnel counseling program in 1936. P. A. Gorman, former president of Western Electric, writes, " 'Personnel Counseling' . . . was an early attempt . . . to implement, to make viable and creative the so-called 'Hawthorne effect' " (Dickson and Roethlisberger 1966, v; Roethlisberger and Dickson 1939). The program, also called "control through listening," assumed that the best way to respond to the workers' irrational behavior and boost their identity with the company was to demonstrate Western Electric's interest in them by listening to their concerns and complaints. The program was staffed by nonprofessionals, most of whom were workers promoted from the shop floor, who wandered through the work areas, chatting with employees and asking how things were going. When they came across an employee they believed needed counseling, they invited the employee back to the office for a confidential talk. The worker spoke of his or her concerns, and the staff member listened sympathetically. Although these conversations were rarely followed up with any changes in the workplace, Western Electric's management and national labor leaders credited personnel counseling with keeping the company union-free in the 1930s and 1940s (Baritz 1961).

Despite the lack of empirical evidence for the human relations theory, its ideas continue to occupy a prominent place in business administration.[1] The dominance of this paradigm can be seen in the number of corporations that currently call their personnel function human resources management (Perrow 1972) and emphasize that good communications give

1. The human relations school has generated a great deal of empirical research and criticism. George Strauss (1969), a student of the human relations school, systematically questioned its assumptions of harmony, need hierarchy, conflict resolution, and participation. Alex Carey and A. J. M. Sykes reexamined the data from the Hawthorne studies and concluded that Roethlisberger and Dickson's conclusions were incorrect: "The results from these studies, far from supporting the various components of the 'human relations approach,' are surprisingly consistent with a rather old-world view about the value of monetary incentives, driving leadership, and discipline" (Carey 1967, 416;

workers a sense of participating in establishing work standards (McGregor 1960; Likert 1967). More recent work experiments, such as the Topeka System (Zwerdling 1980; Jenkins 1973) and job enrichment and enlargement (Freidlander and Brown 1974), also attempt to implement human relations principles by allowing workers limited participation in decisions about how work is to be structured.

Counseling during World War II and the postwar years

During World War II, the all-out war effort produced a shortage of white males with manufacturing experience; consequently, minorities and women with little or no industrial experience were recruited to fill these positions. Hundreds of counseling programs were introduced into the workplace in order to increase war production. These government-supported programs were administered by both management and labor and were meant to help new employees adapt to the discipline of the workplace and to assist white male supervisors, who were uncomfortable supervising women and minorities (Carter 1977). Although the ideology of the human relations school underlay all of them, the programs of that era may be categorized by their objective: social work, mental health, and alcoholism.

Although opposed to management's earlier social welfarism policies on the grounds that they were paternalistic and a substitute for higher wages, the unions nevertheless believed that the social services were important to their members. They simply distrusted management's social welfare workers and wanted the social services under union control (Carter

Sykes 1965). Charles Perrow reviewed the mass of empirical studies produced by the school and concluded "that there is little empirical support for the human relations theory or theories, that extensive efforts to find that support have resulted in increasing limitations and contingencies, and that the grand schemes such as Likert's ['science-based theory'] appear to be methodologically unsound and theoretically biased" (1972, 143).

1977). Consequently, when the labor division of the War Production Board made funds available, the Congress of Industrial Organizations (CIO) initiated a counseling program for its members. This program still exists, and Leo Perlis characterizes it as "the oldest and largest continuing employee assistance program in the country" (1980, 81). More concerned with the health and welfare of the union's membership than with productivity, this unique program relies on rank-and-file workers who are trained to refer fellow workers to community health and social services. Since the program's inception, more than 200,000 union members in more than two hundred communities have been trained as referral agents. In two-hour sessions over a period of eight weeks, they are taught to detect a coworker's problem, to intervene, and to refer the employee to an appropriate agency. These counselors handle a variety of problems from marital discord to money management, from legal aid to alcoholism.

The National Maritime Union's United Seamen's Service was the best known of the union social work programs created during the war. It was developed in 1943 under the leadership of Bertha Capen Reynolds, a pioneer in psychiatric social work. She wrote about the program in her classic, *Social Work and Social Living*:

> The group of social caseworkers . . . were enthusiastic about the opportunity to extend the frontier of social work into a great industry. They saw this as a very different venture from that of counseling in industry as it is sponsored by management. (1975, 58)

There was conflict, however, between the union and the social workers about how to organize the program. The social workers were trained as psychiatric social workers and were prepared to offer such services, while the union members considered their needs to be primarily financial. In particular, the seamen wanted help in securing loans to support their families while they were away fighting the war. Although

13

many of the social workers worried that simply servicing such economic needs would undermine their professional identity and resurrect "the allegation that for this work 'All you need is a kind heart' " (Reynolds 1975, 80), they resolved the conflict in their own favor by using their diagnostic skills to screen loan applicants. These skills were deemed absolutely essential because they permitted the psychiatric social worker to "see through" to the client's "real" needs. For example, when a seaman came to request a loan, the social worker would investigate his emotional and family life and perhaps suggest that a referral to a family services agency and treatment would be more helpful than money. This is not to suggest that none of the seamen and their families benefited from treatment, but it does mean that the psychiatric social workers used their diagnostic skills to decide for the seamen what was in their best interests. Such behavior was in stark contrast to that of both the human relations counselors and the rank-and-file referral agents who listened empathically to the workers' concerns and accepted those concerns at face value.

When the government withdrew its funding at the end of the war, most of the counseling programs closed up shop (Carter 1977). Indeed, the AFL-CIO Community Services was one of the few programs to continue operating, because the union had taken over its funding before the end of the war.

World War II also saw the initiation of psychiatric services in industry. Occupational mental health is concerned with both the psychiatrically ill employee and factors in the work environment that stimulate mentally healthy behavior (McLean 1973, 125). Since the beginning of this century, psychiatrists had been concerned with emotional disturbance and work (e.g., Burlingame 1946, Southard 1920). However, it was the war that brought them out of their consulting rooms and hospital wards in great numbers (Campbell 1943).

During the war, psychiatrists treated emotionally wounded soldiers on the battlefields, generating a theory of stress reaction and its short-term treatment in the process (Daniels 1972). On the homefront, they worked in industry, applying

14

a wide variety of clinical techniques to the prevention and treatment of emotional disturbances. Generally, they believed that emotional problems in industry lie in the individual or in the home or nonwork social surroundings rather than in the job situation (McLean 1973). They used the nondirective counseling techniques pioneered by the Hawthorne studies as well as direct advice (e.g., Gordon 1973) and psychoanalytic therapy. They encouraged industrial physicians, nurses, and supervisors to recognize that employees' emotional problems contributed to high rates of absenteeism, labor turnover, sickness, and low rates of productivity (Rosenbaum and Romano 1943). Employees were most often treated in "emotional first aid stations" (Lott 1946), where, it was argued, a minimum of on-the-job treatment resulted in conspicuous on-the-job improvement (McLean 1973).

It is unclear how many psychiatrists worked in the war industries, and most apparently were employed there only as part-time consultants. In 1943, Dr. George Gehrmann at Dupont was one of the few corporate medical directors to employ one full time. Initially, Dr. F. W. Dershimer was hired under the guise of a general practitioner because Dupont's management refused to have a full-time psychiatrist on its medical staff. Gradually, the other doctors began to refer emotionally disturbed employees to him, and soon he was specializing in psychiatric problems. A year later, Dupont's management agreed to provide for a full-time psychiatrist in the medical budget. Dupont was one of the few companies to continue its psychiatric program after the war ended and most companies closed down their emotional first-aid stations (Ferguson and Fersing, 1965).

After the war, the number of psychiatric programs in industry regrew very slowly. The Vocational Rehabilitation Act of 1943 and the Mental Health Act of 1946 encouraged companies such as Prudential Insurance Company, Caterpillar Tractor, American Cyanamid, and Eastman Kodak to hire psychiatrists and clinical psychologists to rehabilitate psychiatrically handicapped veterans as well as to counsel normal employees (Gordon 1973; Vonachen et al. 1946). Although these programs generally emphasized the prevention and treatment of emotional disturbances, there was no single accepted model for doing so (Ferguson and Fersing 1965; Noland 1973).

Throughout the 1950s, a number of organizations promoted the adoption of occupational mental health programs. The American Psychiatric Association served as a clearinghouse for occupational mental health information, representing the professional viewpoints of the Group for the Advancement of Psychiatry, the American Medical Association, and the Industrial Medical Association (McLean 1973). In 1948, the Cornell University School of Industrial and Labor Relations, under a Carnegie Corporation grant, had begun training psychiatrists to work in industry (Burling and Longaker 1955), and during the 1950s, such diverse groups as the National Training Laboratories, the Menninger Foundation, the University of Cincinnati, and the National Association of Mental Health were also engaged in training psychiatrists, industrial physicians, and executives.

By the mid-sixties, there were approximately a dozen national organizations promoting occupational mental health programs (Ferguson and Fersing 1965). In 1963, Congress passed the Community Mental Health Centers Act, and practitioners hoped that this legislation would lead to a close working relationship between the centers and local businesses (Cohen 1973; McLean 1973). They envisioned the centers as providing outpatient treatment services to employees and as training managers to develop healthy work environments.

Yet the number of occupational mental health programs set up to treat employees remained small. In the mid-1960s, there were approximately two hundred psychiatrists and one hundred fifty clinical psychologists active in industry (McLean 1973). Many of those individuals were working with industry on a part-time basis, performing such prevention tasks as supervisory training, preemployment psychological testing, employee performance appraisal, and psychological research on job satisfaction, morale, and employee attitudes (Ferguson and Fersing 1965). Relatively few psychiatrists and clinical psychologists actually treated employees in the workplace.

In a series of review articles written for the *American Journal of Psychiatry*, F. S. Dershimer (1952, 1953, 1954, 1955) complained about the low regard that managers had for psychiatry. He blamed psychiatrists for this lack of acceptance, stating that they were unrealistic about private enterprise, that they belittled the practical human relations knowledge of industrialists, and that they resorted to name-calling when industry failed to demand their services. In the mid-1960s, several studies (Ferguson and Fersing 1965; Opinion Research Corporation 1966) summarized the current psychiatric thinking about work and mental health, emphasizing the non-psychotic nature of most emotional disturbances in the workplace, and a survey conducted by the Bureau of Business Research at the University of Texas (Mumm and Spiegel 1962) suggested the stubborn resistance of management to occupational mental health programs. The Harvard Business School's report (Ferguson and Fersing 1965) characterized management's disregard as a *Legacy of Neglect* and urged companies to adopt programs as a means of reducing corporate liability for employees' emotional disturbances.

Charles Ferguson and Jan Fersing believed that the occupational mental health movement lacked overall coordination and that until some respected team could plan and promote programs nationally, managers would continue to neglect emotional disturbances in the workplace. Eventually in the early 1970s, a national team, capable of planning and promoting programs, was created by the federal government. It grew, however, out of the occupational alcoholism movement, which developed during the war years separately from the social work and mental health programs. Although encouraged by the personnel shortages, which necessitated hiring and retaining possible alcoholics, these programs were not funded by the federal government. They grew out of the efforts of dedicated members of Alcoholics Anonymous (AA) and

17

corporate physicians who recognized a drinking problem in industry (Trice and Schonbrunn 1981). Among the better known programs of this era were those of Dupont and Eastman Kodak, but such companies as Hudson Department Store of Detroit and Thompson Aircraft Products of Cleveland also developed programs.

The early alcoholism programs were informal arrangements in which there was neither a written company policy nor a program administrator. Usually suspected alcoholics were approached by an AA member who stressed to the suspect that alcoholism was a disease and that recovery was possible through the fellowship. In cases where the alcoholic's job performance was adversely affected by drinking, the AA member stressed that, unless something was done about the drinking, the employee would almost certainly lose his or her job.

Dupont's program, which is considered to be one of the first alcoholism programs in industry (Dunkin 1982), illustrates the close working relationship between physicians and AA members and the manner in which these programs operated. It was created by Dr. George Gehrmann and Dave M. in 1942. Dave M., an AA member, worked at Dupont's Remington Arms Company in Bridgeport, Connecticut, as a personnel adminstrator, where he had become aware of workers with drinking problems. Without the company's knowledge, he approached these employees and induced many of them to join AA. Through fortuitous circumstances, Gehrmann, who had concluded independently that AA could be valuable in treating employees, learned about Dave's work and arranged for him to be transferred to the Delaware headquarters. Here Dave continued to work as a personnel administrator and to approach alcoholic employees informally. In telling an employee about AA, Dave stressed that it was the employee's decision whether to join, but he also emphasized that unless an employee took steps to overcome his or her drinking problem, he or she would probably be discharged for unsatisfactory work performance. Eventually, Dupont formalized this procedure by writing a company policy on alcoholism and by making Dave the first alcoholism counselor in industry.

While the World War II mental health and social work programs expired at the end of the war, the alcoholism programs continued to grow and to become more formalized. This growth can be attributed to the support of AA members, industrial physicians, Yale University's Center of Alcohol Studies,[2] and the National Council on Alcoholism.

The Yale Plan for Business and Industry was directed at teaching business and labor leaders that alcoholism was a treatable disease and that the workplace was the best place to identify and treat the alcoholic. The plan formalized the elements of the World War II programs. It recommended a written policy on alcoholism and the designation of a program coordinator (generally an AA member), and it stressed that supervisors should be taught the signs and symptoms of the disease and how to refer the alcoholic to the program coordinator for counseling and treatment.

For several reasons, the Yale Plan was an important step for industrial alcoholism. First, it put the full weight of prestigious Yale University behind the propositions that alcoholism is a treatable disease and that the workplace is the most effective arena for identifying and treating the alcoholic. Not only was the plan promoted in the prestigious name of Yale University, but it was also based on the research of Yale scientists, which estimated the dollars-and-cents cost of alcoholism to industry (Jellinek 1947; Bacon 1948) and which dispelled the skid-row stereotype of the alcoholic (Bacon 1951). Second, against this backdrop, Lefty Henderson, the program's industrial consultant, developed his "half-man" description and its accompanying rationale for program adoption—it saves money. "Half-man" depicted an employee who was "neither the whole man drunk and obvious, nor the whole man sober

2. Yale's Center of Alcohol Studies was moved to Rutgers University in 1962. For an interesting discussion of Yale's involvement in the alcoholism movement, see Conrad and Schneider (1980a).

and useful" (Henderson and Bacon 1953, 252).[3] Rather, he was the employee who said he "didn't feel up to par" and whose drinking behavior resulted in an average loss of twenty-two working days a year, an inordinate number of visits to the nurse for headaches and stomachaches, and an overuse of disability payments. Half-man's behavior created a hidden cost to the company which could be effectively reduced by adopting the Yale Plan, and in one form or another, this argument has been adopted by occupational consultants ever since.

In 1944, Marty Mann, herself an AA member, founded the National Committee on Education and Alcoholism, which later became known as the National Council on Alcoholism (NCA), to promote the concept of alcoholism as a treatable disease. Since its inception, the Council has maintained a close relationship with the Center of Alcohol Studies, and after Lefty's death in 1958, NCA carried on his work, hiring Lewis Presnall, formerly director of Kennecott Copper's Chino Mines Personnel Counseling Program, to be its industrial consultant. After investigating other companies' programs, Presnall concluded that the majority were ineffective. Drawing on his own experience and on research supported by the Christopher D. Smithers Foundation (e.g., Smithers 1958), he created a new program model, which retained many elements of the Yale Plan (e.g., written policy, program coordinator). Unlike the Yale Plan, however, it stressed that alcoholics could be identified at an earlier stage of their illness if supervisors focused strictly on job performance and stopped relying on such signs as bleary eyes, which are more symptomatic of late-stage alcoholism (Presnall 1966). He also recommended that supervisors confront the employee with his or her deteriorating performance and refer those employees unable to

3. From the 1940s through the 1960s, alcohol programming was directed primarily at male workers. In the 1970s, the emphasis shifted to a more or less equal focus on males and females, due in part to the 1970s influx of women into the workplace and to research claiming that women are as likely to become alcoholic as men are.

correct their performance to the company's counseling program. Although he believed that the majority of problem employees would be alcoholics, Presnall well knew from his Chino Mines experience that focusing on job performance would also identify employees with other personal problems (Presnall 1956, 1966). For this reason, he recommended that programs have a nondiagnostic title, such as "employee counseling service" or "special health services" (Dunkin 1982).

Like their predecessor Lefty Henderson, Lewis Presnall and his colleague Ross Von Wiegand traveled extensively, promoting NCA's new alcoholism program model and the model's effectiveness. Von Wiegand (1971) claims that under the old model 14 to 15 percent of the problem drinkers were motivated to seek treatment but that under the new program model 24 to 76 percent of the problem drinkers were motivated to seek treatment. Although NCA appears to have been very successful in promoting its new programs, its leaders believed that its diffusion was too slow.

> The most important factor which has prevented utilization of the new approach is that most American employer organizations are not aware of the development of the new approach, nor its simplicity and effectiveness. (Von Wiegand 1971)

That was about to change.

Encouraged by the community mental health movement's success in acquiring government support, the emerging alcoholism industry vigorously lobbied the federal government to establish a separate institute for the study of alcoholism (Trice and Roman 1978, Wiener 1981). The individuals and organizations who made up the industry argued that alcoholism is not a mental illness per se and requires alternative approaches to prevention, identification, and treatment.

The alcoholism constituency was successful in pressuring the federal government to appropriate funds. Because the federal government, working toward President Johnson's vision of the Great Society, had appropriated money for other social and health problems, it became increasingly difficult for legislators to do less in the case of alcoholism. More important, the alcoholism constituency had very powerful allies in Congress, a cadre of legislators who were members of AA and believed that the only way to have alcoholism fully accepted as a disease by the American public was to put the weight of the federal government behind it. Led by Senator Harold Hughes of Iowa, this group cajoled their fellow senators and representatives into passing the Comprehensive Alcohol Abuse and Alcoholism Prevention and Treatment Act of 1970, the Hughes Act, which established the National Institute on Alcohol Abuse and Alcoholism (NIAAA).

NIAAA's Division of Special Treatment and Rehabilitation Programs created an occupational alcoholism programs branch. Its efforts emphasized that alcoholism was the prevalent problem among workers and that constructive confrontation was essential in identifying the hidden alcoholic. NIAAA called its approach the Employee Assistance Program (EAP) in order to establish an identity separate from NCA.

In order to promote EAPs to American employers, NIAAA funded and trained two occupational program consultants (OPCs) in each state. The states did the recruiting, and each state used its own criteria for recruitment. Consequently, the majority of occupational program consultants had little academic, professional, or personal experience with alcoholism treatment or with the fellowship of AA (Roman and Trice 1976). Many were mental health specialists, and they split the consultants' group into two opposing camps. Those OPCs who were involved with the alcoholism industry stressed both that alcoholism was the major health problem in the workplace and that supervisory referrals were the most effective means of identifying the potential alcoholic. Those OPCs who were mental health specialists stressed that all problems were equally important and that the best way to reach these troubled employees was to encourage them to refer themselves.

The battle raged until 1975. NCA and the Community Services Department of the AFL-CIO advocated the alcohol approach. The AFL-CIO opposed the mental health model as a potentially unlimited mechanism of social control that could be abused by management and as a competitor with its union counseling program. The matter was publicly debated at the 1975 meeting of the Association of Labor-Management Administrators and Consultants on Alcoholism (ALMACA), where the ALMACA leaders pleaded for an end to the divisiveness and for some consensus (Roman 1981a). It was uneasily conceded that work organizations should determine the form and label of their own programs.

Although the NCA and the AFL-CIO continue to express periodic opposition to the mental health approach, the mental health version of the EAP is widespread (Trice and Beyer 1981b; Roman 1981a). According to Paul Roman's Executive Caravan Study (1982), 57 percent of the companies surveyed had programs for the identification and assistance of employees with alcohol problems. Sixty-two percent of those programs were part of a broader employee assistance program. In companies with alcoholism intervention programs but without employee assistance programs, 62 percent of the respondents indicated a desire for the broader program. Seven percent of the respondents reported that their companies had employee assistance programs that did not include a component for alcohol problems.

Program growth in the seventies

The number of work organizations reporting that they have emotional health programs has grown tremendously since the early 1970s. Before 1970, there were probably no more than several hundred companies offering programs to their employees, and the bulk of those were focused on alcoholism. It is unclear how many programs currently exist in the United States. ALMACA claims there are approximately twenty-five hundred (Byers 1979), while an article in the *EAP Digest* estimates there are five thousand (Witti 1980), and some enthusiasts calculate as many as ten thousand. Paul Roman (1982), reviewing longitudinal data collected for the Executive Caravan Surveys from 1972 to 1979, found that the percentage of Fortune 500 companies and leading banking, insurance, utilities, transportation, and financial corporations claiming to have programs increased from 25 percent in 1972 to 56 percent in 1979. The Washington Business Group on Health predicts that corporate mental wellness programs are destined to become a major form for the delivery of mental health services (Goldbeck 1979).

Their proliferation has created intense occupational conflict for new program positions. Social workers, alcoholism specialists, and psychologists all claim that their group is best equipped to manage programs and treat troubled employees, and each occupation is gearing up to train its members for emotional health programs. Industrial psychiatrists, long silent on the subject of programs, have responded to these activities by stating that none of these groups has the necessary organizational or clinical skills to practice in the workplace, and they appear poised to assert their legal mandate over the delivery of all psychiatric and medical services. Nevertheless, ALMACA is developing national standards for all practitioners, regardless of their occupational allegiance, and hopes to have a certification process in place soon.

At the same time, the proliferation of emotional health programs has created opportunities for entrepreneurs interested in providing outside treatment services to employees. In 1981, Roman (1981a) estimated that there were approximately two hundred such private groups in the country. Although no one knows exactly how large this group and its revenues are, by all accounts it is growing. In New York City, for example, where only the NCA was delivering such services in 1970, there are at least a dozen profit-seeking agencies (several with offices throughout the United States) devoted solely to providing diagnostic and treatment services to emotional health programs. An indication of the amount of money to be made from such services is the National Employee Assistance Providers Association (NEAPA), a trade association formed in 1981 by ten companies that provide treatment services to emotional health programs. NEAPA's purpose is to promote the special interests of private, profit-seeking groups, and its first priority is to bar mental health centers that receive federal or state funding from providing diagnostic and treatment services to occupational programs. It is NEAPA's position that these organizations have an unfair competitive advantage:

> While recognizing the pioneering efforts of the public sector in EAP development, our members believe that the future of the EAP field lies in the hands of entrepreneurs who have risked capital to compete in this new and challenging field. They believe that within the free enterprise system lies the highest level of accountability, thus the highest level of care for the troubled employee. (Hellan 1981)

On the basis of these remarks, it seems fair to conclude that emotional health programs have become big business, and that such turf fights will probably continue.

There are a number of reasons for the corporate trend toward adopting emotional health programs, but primarily, managers adopt them because they believe that helping employees solve their personal problems is good business (Roman 1982; Trice and Beyer 1984a). This belief, which combines concerns for compassion and productivity, is reflected in social welfarism and human relations, and managers who support these philosophies are more likely than are those who believe in social Darwinism or scientific management to adopt programs. Several factors have influenced management belief in compassion and emotional health programs: government support, escalating health care costs, corporate liability for work stress, and the society's tendency to make troublesome behavior a medical problem.

The federal government contributed directly to the growth of emotional health programs by establishing NIAAA and

25

funding occupational program consultants. By all indications, the national network of OPCs has been enormously successful in its marketing efforts, indeed, so successful that, when their original funding expired, a majority of the states continued to support their marketing efforts under the states' budgets. Another measure of success is the variety of organizations and occupations currently imitating the occupational program consultants. If imitation is the sincerest form of flattery, it is also the surest sign of success in the business world.

In addition, the federal government contributed indirectly to program adoption by creating agencies that limited management's control, for instance, the Equal Employment Opportunities Commission, Civil Rights Commission, and Federal Contracts Compliance Office. Such authors as William G. Scott and David K. Hart (1979) and Richard Edwards (1979) have commented on the manner in which such federal agencies limited management's discretion to discipline employees and prompted them to search for new methods to control workers. The adoption of an emotional health program is one such alternative; indeed, the occupational program consultants marketed treatment programs as an effective means of controlling employees with personal problems. The research of Trice and his colleagues indicates that companies that adopt programs perceive the programs "as helping supervisors manage marginally performing employees" (1981, 312; see also Trice and Beyer 1984a), and indeed while I was working as a consultant, a vice president of human resources for a Fortune 500 Company remarked to me,

> We need some way to handle these difficult cases. We have got this black woman who thinks she should be a general manager because of all this affirmative action stuff. She is not a terrific performer, and we do not dare fire her for fear of a lawsuit. Maybe the counseling program can straighten her out.

Usually executives are not so explicit about using the program to cool out employees, but his comments reflect the concerns of many managers with whom I have discussed program development over the past eleven years.

In a similar manner, arbitration cases have limited the ability of managers to discipline employees with alcohol, drug, and emotional troubles (Denenberg and Denenberg 1983; Shain and Walden 1980). For instance, progressive disciplinary procedures that do not include an offer of therapeutic help are being increasingly regarded by arbitrators as inadequate. Accordingly,

> Employee Assistance Programs have a large role to play in affording an alcoholic [an addict or emotionally disturbed employee] an opportunity for recovery. Their role should be recognized in the arbitration process, and "due process" arguments which might thwart their proper functioning should be scrutinized carefully. Ideally, no discharge case should arrive at the arbitration stage before there has been an effort to have the Employee Assistance Program deal with the problems which underlie the behavior that led to the discipline. (Denenberg and Denenberg 1983, 144)

It is no secret that the costs of health care are rising at astronomical rates. As costs increase, so do the insurance premiums paid by employers. Occupational program consultants contended that program adoption would significantly reduce premiums by ensuring that alcoholism was properly diagnosed and treated as such rather than as some other disease, for instance, a gastrointestinal disorder (Wrich 1974 and 1980). At the same time that the consultants were marshaling evidence to prove their case, medical researchers began to compile evidence demonstrating that such chronic diseases as heart disease and cancer that were driving up health costs could be prevented.

The Washington Business Group on Health has developed and marketed their mental-wellness programs on this diverse information. With 160 Fortune 500 Companies on its membership roster, the group emphasizes corporate social responsibility for reducing health care costs by developing company programs for the prevention and early diagnosis of emotional and physical problems. Based on survey data from sixty-eight companies with programs, the group concluded,

> The potential for good return on investment in mental wellness is substantial. If only a small percentage of the otherwise unnecessary utilization of hospital/surgical/medical benefits is eliminated, the programs will pay for themselves. (Kiefhaber and Goldbeck 1980, 26)

Speaking at the 1978 Conference on Employee Mental Wellness, Walter Wriston, former chairman of Citicorp, concurred:

> An individual patient may have little leverage on the kind and the cost of medical care available, but employers of large numbers of people do have an opportunity and an obligation to determine what health care is wanted and to design reimbursement formulas accordingly. If the private sector does not act constructively to design programs to contain medical costs at a level consistent with quality care, then the government will step in with the kind of cost controls that invariably erode incentives for quality. . . . We must do so without bankrupting our companies or the nation. (1980, ix)

It is difficult to know what proportion of companies have actually adopted programs because of these exhortations, but it is my impression that many of the companies that adopt programs do so with the hope of reducing future health care costs.

Corporate liability for stress-related disability is another strong influence in the proliferation of emotional health programs. On September 17, 1980, the *Wall Street Journal* published a news article titled "On-the-Job Stress Leads Many Workers to File—and Win—Compensation Awards" (Lublin 1980). The newspaper was immediately deluged with requests for reprints. What stimulated such corporate interest? The article documented a startling increase in disability payments for severe anxiety, depression, and other mental problems caused by work stress and stated that the trend might fuel demands for legislative overhaul of the workers' compensation system. Before the Michigan Supreme Court's decision in *Carter* v. *General Motors Corporation* in 1960, compensation laws limited claims primarily to physical injury. But in this case, the court awarded Carter disability compensation based on traumatic neurosis and psychosis that developed over the course of his employment because of the extreme demands made upon him by his supervisor (Blum 1980). Courts in at least six other states have ruled that emotionally ill employees deserve awards for stress accumulated on the job. In California, where in 1971 the State Supreme Court upheld compensation for such cases, officials estimate that they receive at least three to four thousand psychiatric-injury claims a year and that about half of the distressed workers receive awards (Lublin 1980). Such developments prompted the Washington Business Group on Health to advise corporations,

> Mental wellness programs are rapidly becoming a legal responsibility rather than a matter of choice. The implications of state and federal trends should be obvious. The more that employers can do now to demonstrate a willingness to provide effective means of dealing with these health problems, the less pressure there will be for more regulations. (Kiefhaber and Goldbeck 1979, 19–20)

While it is unclear what proportion of companies have actually adopted programs on the basis of such concerns, evidence from alcoholism research suggests that the stress issue has always been an important factor in program adoption. Harrison Trice and Paul Roman (1978) clearly documented the stressful work factors that contribute to the development of alcoholism. Although occupational program consultants have never used this etiological data as a rationale for program development (Roman and Trice 1976), the consultants have told executives that the presence of a program would aid them

29

in difficult court cases with aggrieved alcoholic employees—
a claim substantially borne out in the regular reprints on
compensation cases issued by NCA's *Labor-Management Alcoholism Journal*. One rationale for program adoption is that
treatment helps erase the harmful effects of stress and assists
the company to protect its liability, and when a program has
been adopted, stress education has generally been part of the
program's focus. For example, in *The Employee Assistance
Program*, James Wrich quotes an educational pamphlet titled
Stress:

> How do you handle stressful situations? . . . Stress and
> tension are common occurrences in everyday living. . . .
> How do I know if I need professional help? . . . Your Em-
> ployee Assistance Program can help you decide what
> might be the best for you and your family . . . .(1980, 195)

International Paper Company's EAP distributes a pamphlet
on stress that contains the Holmes-Rahe life stress test (Holmes
and Rahe 1967) and encourages employees with high scores
to seek professional help; and stress management seminars
have become a regular feature at ALMACA meetings. Considering the stress emphasis in programs and the increasing
liability to companies for illnesses induced by on-the-job stress,
it does not seem unreasonable to assume that these factors
have contributed and will continue to contribute to program
adoption.

Underlying all the other phenomena that have contributed
to the increasing number of emotional health programs is the
general tendency of society to make a medical problem of
troublesome behavior. Peter Conrad and Joseph Schneider
(1980a) demonstrate persuasively that a wide variety of social
behaviors considered troublesome have come under the ju-
risdiction of the medical and paramedical establishments. The
United States' culture, which emphasizes individualism, humanitarianism, pragmatism, and science, provided a fertile
ground for the growth of scientific medicine and its medical
model. Interest groups, such as AA and the National Mental

Health Association, and physician activists pressured local, state, and federal legislatures to pass laws making such behaviors medical problems and to provide funds for their treatment by medical personnel. The process by which personal problems come to be seen as troublesome and are referred to corporate treatment as a medical problem is considered in the pages that follow.

2. Trouble and emotional health programs

Troubles often begin as a vague sense of "something wrong." As people try to understand what is the matter and what to do about it, they come to define the trouble as a particular kind of problem: alcoholism, schizophrenia, depression, marital difficulties. People arrive at such definitions by seeking and receiving advice from others and by trying different remedies to control the difficulty. In some cases, people try to remedy the problem themselves by trying harder or doing better; in other cases, friends or family members at first cajole and later insist that they take some course of action. Still, in other situations, the police, a doctor, or some other authority may intercede, casting the troublemakers off to jail or treatment. If this happens, the troublemakers may come to perceive of themselves as alcoholics, schizophrenics, depressives, wife beaters, or whatever. Troubles, then, have a natural history: the interactional processes through which personal difficulties are identified, reacted to, elaborated, and transformed into a particular kind of problem (Emerson and Messinger 1977).

There is nothing inherent in any behavior or condition that makes it troublesome; rather it becomes defined as troublesome when one group tries to impose its standards upon another. For instance, playing a stereo is not inherently troublesome; however, when adults and teenagers, who have different standards of music and tolerances for loudness, interact, it can quickly become a problem. The adults will attempt to make the youngsters turn down the volume on their stereos, and the teenagers will try to avoid doing so. In a similar manner, airlines attempt to impose their weight regulations upon stewardesses; companies insist upon certain dress codes; and the military enforces restrictions on facial hair.

Definitions of trouble vary with social context. For example, outside a nudist camp, nudity enjoys little social support (Weinberg 1978). Consequently, the man who parades naked down Fifth Avenue in New York City most likely will be arrested for being an exhibitionist and either thrown in jail or admitted to Bellevue Hospital for psychiatric care. On the other hand, the fully clad man in a nudist colony may become identified as a peeping Tom and trespasser, arrested, and given psychotherapy for his voyeurism.

Definitions of trouble emerge from the remedies used by individuals and groups to control the perceived shortcomings of others. For instance, in trying to control someone's disruptive drinking behavior a variety of solutions may be imposed. His wife may try to control it by pouring his bottles down the sink; his friends may shun him; the police may arrest and send him to DWI classes; and his employer might send him to an alcoholism rehabilitation program. Such cures are imposed upon the drinker provisionally and, if one is found to work, the trouble is defined within that particular context. If the DWI classes correct his disruptive behavior, he will become defined as a problem drinker who with a little punishment and education is able to resume drinking. If the rehabilitation works, he will become defined as an alcoholic who abstains from alcohol and joins Alcoholics Anonymous. If those remedies fail, other solutions will be sought. Defining trouble then is a fluid social process, and the cures brought to bear upon a particular difficulty have social consequences for everyone involved.

In remedying trouble, people use self-control as well as relational and formal social controls. People exercise self-control when they recognize the beginnings of trouble in themselves and stop themselves from deviating from group standards. They are said to have a conscience and are willing to try harder. The stewardess who keeps her weight down and the soldier who maintains a short, neat haircut exercise self-control and are not troublesome. Relational controls are interactions between individuals that positively or negatively sanction a behavior. Relational controls include ridicule, praise, gossip, smiles, disapproving looks, ostracism, and social support. When the stewardess's coworkers tease her about gaining a few extra pounds and when the business executive's co-workers compliment her on the cut and color of her suit, their co-workers are exercising relational controls. These controls both inhibit individuals from behavior that might be considered troublesome and encourage conformity by positive sanctions.

When self-control and relational controls fail to remedy trouble, people resort to formal social controls. Formal controls reside in social institutions that operate, explicitly and implicitly, to secure adherence to a particular set of values and norms. The education, criminal justice, welfare, and medical systems perform social control functions. Crime and illness are both designations for trouble. Broadly speaking, the criminal justice system punishes individuals for troublesome behavior that is perceived as willful, and the medical system treats individuals for troublesome behavior that is seen as involuntary. Criminals are punished with the goal of altering their behavior to create conformity; sick people are treated with the goal of altering the conditions that prevent their conformity.

Historically, there has been a general trend away from punishing people as troublemakers to treating them as troubled individuals. Consequently, many behaviors, formerly regarded as normal, sinful, or criminal have been labeled as illnesses and brought within medicine's domain. This domain includes physicians and psychiatrists as well as such limited health practitioners as clinical psychologists, psychiatric social workers, and alcohol and drug counselors. In treating troublesome behaviors, medical practitioners use a wide range of technologies, including drugs, surgery, behavior modifications, and genetic screening (Conrad and Schneider 1980a). Tranquilizers are prescribed for anxiety, nervousness, and general malaise; methodone is prescribed for heroine addiction; and amphetamines are prescribed for overeating and obesity. Behavior modification has been used to treat mental illness, homosexuality, violence, autism, phobias, alcoholism, and drug addiction.

The medical system exercises social control through its ability to confer the sick role, a process intended to return sick persons to their normal social roles and minimize the disruption illness causes in society (Parsons 1951; Freidson 1970). The person cast in the sick role is exempted from normal responsibilities, at least to the extent necessary to get well, is not held responsible for his or her condition, and cannot be expected to recover by an act of will. In return, the sick person must recognize that being ill is an inherently undesirable state, must want to recover, and is obligated to seek and cooperate with a competent treatment agent.

Any social setting generates a number of ambiguous difficulties. As we have seen, these difficulties may ultimately be—but are not immediately—identified as troublesome. Social research examines how, within a particular setting, self-control and relational and formal controls are brought to bear upon these vague difficulties so that they become identified and organized into a specific kind of trouble. For example, Marian Yarrow and her colleagues (1955) examined the processes by which wives tried to control the bizarre behavior of their husbands who were later diagnosed as mentally ill. Generally, they could not remember when or how the troubles first started but were able to recount how they tried to control the difficulties by prodding and threatening their husbands and by making elaborate excuses for them. Consequently, they were able to think of their husbands' behavior as normal until outside authorities intervened. Once this happened, however, they began to perceive of their husbands as mentally ill. Other researchers have studied the negotiation processes by which vague difficulties are transformed into a specific kind of trouble in college psychiatric service (Schwartz and Kahne 1977, 1983; Kahne and Schwartz 1978), an outpatient drug treatment program (Peyrot 1985), a battered women's shelter (Ferraro 1983), and nursing homes (Diamond 1983).

Trouble and work organizations

Emotional health programs, which are embedded in work organizations' control structures, have taken two approaches to trouble, disciplinary and medical. Older alcoholism programs transformed employees' troubles into disciplinary issues by constructively confronting problem drinkers about their unsatisfactory job performance. Under these circumstances, it was assumed that the majority of problem drinkers could control their own drinking and improve their performance. Employees were assumed to suffer from an illness only if they were unable to improve their performance.

Constructive confrontation evolved as a technique for overcoming two problems: the difficulty of identifying employed alcoholics and the reluctance of supervisors to confront employees about their problem drinking (Trice and Roman 1978). Alcoholism is a progressive disorder, and in its middle stages, it is difficult to distinguish problem drinkers from alcoholic employees because those who are merely abusing alcohol as well as those who are addicted to it are likely to get into trouble on the job, at home, or in the community. This is made doubly difficult because alcoholics, when faced with the untoward consequences of their drinking behavior, will deny that there is anything wrong.

Supervisors usually know when employees are having problems with their drinking because they either drink with them or hear gossip about their troubles from family members or coworkers. They also become aware of the drinking problems when employees' job performance begins to deteriorate, which typically occurs during the middle stages of alcoholism. Supervisors, however, are reluctant to confront the problem drinkers because in American society there are powerful norms against interfering in other people's personal affairs and because they fear being blamed and held responsible for employees' poor performance. Consequently, supervisors vascillate in seeing the employee's behavior as troublesome and often delay confronting employees until their disease has progressed into late-stage alcoholism.

Constructive confrontation solves the problem of identifying alcoholic employees by adopting a pragmatic definition of alcoholism based upon job performance. "Normal drinking" is drinking that does not unduly alter behavior and does not interfere with effective and efficient work performance. "Problem drinking" is behavior that *both* exceeds the bounds of community definitions and impairs job performance. "Alcohol addiction" is defined as physiological loss of control over drinking and is generally indicated by employees' inability to control their drinking and maintain an acceptable level of job performance. These definitions use job performance as a criterion for identifying problem drinkers and alcoholics, and they assume that those employees who are merely abusing alcohol can be motivated to change their behavior and that those who have lost control of their drinking will be motivated to seek medical treatment. Constructive confrontation supplies this motivation.

Constructive confrontation prescribes that supervisors hold a number of discussions with employees whose performance is unacceptable. During the initial discussion, supervisors confront employees with evidence of their impaired performance and offer assistance for rehabilitation in a constructive manner. In the confrontational part of the discussion, the employees are given feedback on the specifics of unacceptable work performance and warned that continued unacceptable performance is likely to lead eventually to formal discipline. In the constructive part, supervisors remind employees that practical assistance is available from the alcoholism program. Subsequent steps in the intervention depend on the response of employees. If performance improves, nothing happens; if unacceptable performance continues, several more informal discussions may follow. At all times, however, employees are free to choose whether or not to go to the program for help. The constructive part of such informal discussions (1) expresses emotional support and group concern about the employee's welfare; (2) emphasizes that group membership can be maintained if the employee conforms better in the future; and (3) suggests that an alternative course of behaviors that the employee can take is available to regain satisfactory work performance. The confrontational part of such discussions (1) reiterates internalized values upheld by the group (in this case, expectations of work performance); (2) reminds employees that they are not fulfilling these expectations and that sanctions will follow if expectations continue to be violated; and (3) establishes some social distance between the employee and those group members who are meeting expectations, thus setting the stage for further sanctions, if needed.

Eventually, if the employee's performance still does not improve, management uses a supplementary tactic called "crisis precipitation," in which the employee is formally disciplined for continued poor performance—initially with a written warning, then with a series of increasingly long temporary suspensions, and finally with discharge. Like any discipline used in attempts at social control, the progressively more severe sanctions embodied in the disciplinary steps of job-based programs are intended to make the personal cost of troublesome behavior so high that the person will be motivated to stop and to deter others from similar behaviors.

Research suggests that constructive confrontation is effective. Supervisors who are properly trained and who are also integrated into an informal supervisory network that supports the strategy have little difficulty in implementing it (Belasco and Trice 1969; Googins and Kurtz 1981). Indeed, the most important determinant of whether supervisors use constructive confrontation is the support that they receive from other supervisors, co-workers, and union representatives (Beyer et al. 1980; Kurtz et al., 1980; Roman 1981b). Problem drinkers faced with the possibility of increasingly more severe sanctions are likely to improve their job performance on their own, and alcoholic employees confronted with the probability of job loss and the possibility of rehabilitation are usually motivated to accept help and improve their performance (Trice and Beyer 1984b).

> Constructive confrontation avoids using disease labels as much as possible. Based as it is on the legitimate relationship between the employee and the employer, confrontation can be based on the existence of inappropriate behavior without attributing disease. Medical labeling and treatment is the last step, used when it is evident that the [trouble] is out of the individual's control, that a genuine sickness exists, and that he is unable to respond to confrontation. (Trice and Roman 1978, 174–75)

In programs that have broadened their focus to include emotional, marital, financial, and other personal problems and offer the services of psychiatrists, psychologists, and social workers, constructive confrontation is down played, and self-referral is emphasized.

> Voluntarism . . . is indicative of a successful EAP [employee assistance program] and should be a goal of such a program. (Wrich 1974, 43)

This change in emphasis occurred because mental health professionals are less enthusiastic than are their alcoholism counterparts about any use of discipline and because they believe in the need for treatment or counseling for all personal problems. By emphasizing self-referral, newer emotional health programs bypass the disciplinary process and transform *all* employee troubles into some form of medical problem. This shift from supervisory to medical expertise for solving employees' troubles is referred to as medicalization (Roman 1980). Trice and Beyer call it the "rush to treatment" (1984a).

39

Factors influencing self-referral

Despite the increasing number of emotional health programs and the shift in emphasis from constructive confrontation to self-referral, no one has studied the natural history of troubles that employees voluntarily bring to programs. Consequently, little is known about how employees come to see themselves as troubled, how they decide voluntarily to go to the emotional health program, and what happens to them when they get there. In the following chapters, I attempt to close this research gap by presenting an empirical study of one company's program. However, before doing so, I shall briefly review the research on utilization of medical facilities outside the workplace for clues as to how employees decide to refer themselves to a program. John McKinlay (1972) identifies several important factors that motivate individuals to use medical services outside the workplace: economic, geographic, sociopsychological, and sociocultural.

Research shows that, even when financial costs are removed, wide variations in use of medical services still remain among income and ethnic groups (Kadushin 1967; Suchman 1965). Even with Medicaid and Medicare, low-income groups remain underserved (Aday 1975). On the other hand, Richard Kulka and his colleagues (1979; see also Veroff et al. 1981) state that the gap between the use of psychotherapy by lower and that of upper income groups is decreasing. They attribute this decrease to the availability of Medicare and Medicaid coverage of psychiatric problems. Nevertheless, the issue of insurance coverage is important only after the potential client has recognized the problem as appropriate for psychotherapy. Before that moment, social, psychological, and cultural factors determine whether an individual will see his or her troubles as a mental health problem and decide to seek help. For example, Melvin Glasser and his associates (1975) found that United Auto Workers and their referral agents (e.g., union officials, clergy) were less likely than were mental health professionals to define behaviors and conditions as requiring mental health treatment and that this difference in perspective was a major obstacle to the use of the United Auto Workers' prepaid insurance plan.

Research provides conflicting evidence about whether proximity to health services alone influences their use. Alan Jacobson and his colleagues (1978) studied a Boston neighborhood health center that served a predominantly white, Irish-American, working-class community and a small enclave of professionals. They concluded that, when mental health services are provided in an integrated delivery system near the patient's home, the mental health services may achieve high levels of acceptability, accessibility, and utilization. On the other hand, Harold Luft and his colleagues' (1976) research in rural Livingston, California, found that income, travel time, and price were unimportant in considering medical utilization and that the most important determinant of use was whether individuals felt their health status was in jeopardy. In a study of black adolescents in central Harlem, Ann Brunswick and her colleagues (1979) found that the best predictors of health care use were the person's private physician and a mother born outside the South, and they conclude psychological, social and cultural influences are better predictors of health care use than is the availability of services.

The social-psychological research incorporates the concepts of motivation (people behave to satisfy needs), perception (people behave in accord with the way they perceive the world), and learning (people behave as a function of what is learned) as the major determinants in utilization of services (e.g., Fabrega 1973; Kosa and Robertson 1969; Mechanic 1968; Rosenstock 1966; Suchman 1965; Zola 1964). Marshall Becker (1979) has combined the ideas of these researchers into the health belief model. People who exhibit the appropriate combination of motives and beliefs will accept and undertake recommended behaviors designed to prevent illness while asymptomatic, to define the state of their health in the presence of symptoms, and to restore health after diagnosis of actual illness. Highly suggestive, the model does not explain the origins of beliefs or the conditions under which they are acquired, and it tends to portray the decision to use a service as a static rather than a dynamic process of interaction with individuals, groups, and organizations. Although several authors have suggested various stages in the decision to use a service, relatively little is known about the social factors that affect this process. Furthermore, the inverse of the health belief model is equally likely, that having decided to use a program produces certain beliefs and attitudes.

Socio-cultural research attempts to answer some of the questions raised by the social-psychological approach by placing utilization within a broader cultural setting and within a larger social structure (Zola 1966 and 1973; Suchman 1964 and 1966; Freidson 1961 and 1970). This literature states that people's reactions to symptoms are based upon the definitions provided by their culture, reference group, or social class.

Eliot Freidson's concept of the lay referral system (1961, 1970) illustrates the socio-cultural approach and demonstrates the control consumers exercise over professional medical practice. It states that whether or not individuals will define themselves as ill and decide to refer themselves to a professional is a function of the lay referral system's congruence with the professional culture and of the cohesiveness of the interrelationships of the laypersons from whom advice and referral are sought. Individual's reactions to symptoms are based on the knowledge that they possess. The knowledge of the lay referral network may or may not be in agreement with that of medical professionals, but the more similarity between these groups, the greater the probability that individuals will refer themselves to the medical system. Individuals from tightly knit communities are less inclined to consult with others outside the community than are individuals from less tightly knit ones. Therefore, individuals in a tightly knit community whose health knowledge does not agree with the professional medical culture will be less likely to use professional medical care than will individuals in a less tightly knit community whose health knowledge is congruent with the professional medical culture.

Several other researchers use concepts analogous to the lay referral network (e.g., Scheff 1966, Hawkins and Tiedeman 1975). Charles Kadushin (1969) speaks of contact with the "friends and supporters of psychotherapy" as the most important variable in determining whether people go to a psychiatrist. These friends help individuals to think of their problems as ones requiring psychotherapy and provide advice on referrals to psychotherapists and treatment agencies.

Allan Horwitz's study of a mental health center (1977) suggests how relationships in the workplace affect the decisions of males and females to seek psychotherapy. According to Horwitz, women are more likely than men to discuss their problems with family, friends, and co-workers. This difference in help-seeking behavior leads men and women along two different paths to psychotherapy: women are more likely to seek help voluntarily, and men are more likely to be pressured into it. Women may tentatively label their problem psychiatric and discuss it with others who confirm the label and suggest a referral to a psychotherapist. Or they may discuss their problem with others and accept a suggested psychiatric label and a referral to a psychotherapist. Men, because they are less likely to discuss their problems with others, are more likely than women to have a psychiatric label and referral to a psychotherapist forced upon them. In general, their families and employers coerce them into seeing a psychotherapist when the men's behaviors disrupt the household or the workplace. Whereas women experience work as a place to seek help for their problems, men experience it as an involuntary display area for their symptoms. Horwitz concludes that both culture and social control functions influence labeling and help-seeking patterns. When socialization is weak, social controls are invoked to pressure individuals into treatment.

Margaret Heyman (1976, 1978) makes a similar observation about alcoholic employees referred to industrial alcoholism programs. Alcoholics participate in drinking cultures that actively support their behavior and discourage voluntary referral to treatment. She identifies five triggering incidents that prompted the employees to seek help. In each case, the employee was being coerced by someone at work or in the family to go for help. She concluded, "It is highly doubtful that an alcoholic ever comes to an alcoholism program in industry on a truly voluntary basis" (1976, 907). Other observers (Freedburg and Johnston 1979; Schramm et al. 1978) have reached similar conclusions about alcoholic employees.

Beyond these insights, there remain the puzzling questions of why employees voluntarily risk being stigmatized as mentally ill by their employers and what are the social consequences of using an emotional health program. Indeed, many employees pay their own psychiatric fees rather than use their mental health insurance coverage because they fear what will happen if their employers discover they are seeing a psychotherapist. As a young worker explained to a *New York Times* reporter,

> I have been thinking about using my psychiatric benefits to pay for my treatment. I'd rather pay cash, although I don't have much money, and this is a sacrifice. I have taken a computer course and know that anyone with a terminal can get my record simply by punching in the right code. I am taking a business course now and have learned what lengths some companies go to in order to investigate employees. I must consider my future. I have the ambition one day to go into politics. (Sobel 1981, C1–2)

Longitudinal data show that although individuals in 1976 were more willing to consider professional help for their personal problems than were individuals in 1957, "in both survey years, about one out of seven people who were presumably ready for such help refused to go because of what others might think" (Veroff et al. 1981, 197).[1]

1. Joan Brockman and her colleagues (1979) suggest that the increasingly

The research problem

Although the research on utilization of medical facilities illuminates many aspects of a person's decision to use mental health services, it says little about the natural history of employees' troubles in emotional health programs, that is, the workplace processes that assist them in defining their difficulties as medical problems and the social consequences of voluntarily bringing their difficulties to the program. The remainder of this book examines these questions with the use of empirical observations of one company's emotional health program. The following chapter describes the research setting and field methods used to collect and analyze the data. Chapter 4 examines the process by which employees learn to see their troubles as medical problems and decide to refer themselves to the emotional health program. Chapter 5 examines the ways in which emotional health programs diagnose and treat employees' troubles, and chapter 6 looks at the social consequences of treating employees' troubles as medical problems.

positive public attitude toward the mentally ill is largely an artifact of research methodology. Medical professionals, who prefer using closed-ended interviews, tend to find positive public attitudes toward the mentally ill; however, social scientists, who prefer using open-ended interviews with vignettes or closed-ended self-response questionnaires, tend to find negative public attitudes toward the mentally ill.

3. Corpco and its employees: the fieldwork

Doing fieldwork entails participating in the ongoing activities of a group's life for a considerable length of time, observing events as they unfold, and understanding the meaning that group members attach to those activities and events (Denzin 1978; Patton 1980; Spradley 1979; Whyte 1984). These features make fieldwork an excellent method for studying the natural history of the troubles employees voluntarily bring to the emotional health program because they allow the researcher to understand how people interpret what happens to them and observe how those interpretations change in response to events. Field methods yield "thick descriptions" (Geertz 1973) from which researchers generate hypotheses and theory; they are not used to test hypotheses, which is the function of statistical and experimental methods.

The purposes of this field study were to generate a description and theory about how employees' troubles are transformed into medical problems in one company's emotional health program. In particular, I was interested in understanding how employees decide to refer themselves to the program and what happens to them when they do. Participant observation, document analysis, and in-depth interviews were used to collect data on these processes, and I used the constant comparative method to generate and provisionally test the generated theory (Glaser and Strauss 1967). The constant comparative method is an analytic strategy for generating and plausibly suggesting many properties and hypotheses about a general phenomenon and is used for discovering theory. It cannot be used for testing theory because the collected data are coded only enough to generate, hence, to suggest theory that closely fits one's field observations. Theory generated by this strategy usually cannot be completely refuted by more data or replaced by another theory because it is too intimately linked to the original data. It is destined to last despite its inevitable modification and reformulation. At the same time, the theory is sufficiently developed so that researchers can operationalize it for rigorous testing by statistical methods and practitioners can apply it to their programs.

Gaining access to Corpco

Although there is a growing literature on emotional health programs, the bulk of it consists of articles written to support the ideological stances of mental health practitioners and alcoholism specialists and to convince management of the values of program implementation, and only a small portion is based on empirical observations in work settings. This dearth of research stems from the difficulty of obtaining access to work settings, given the tendency of employers to be secretive.

My own experience in locating a site to conduct this research bore out the experience of other researchers. I approached twenty-four companies in the New York metropolitan area about obtaining access to their programs and employee populations. Twenty-three declined to participate because company policies routinely denied access to outside researchers, because the companies were undergoing a reorganization, or because administrators feared the research would compromise employee confidentiality or were too busy.

Consequently, the research was conducted in the one company that did agree to participate, an organization I shall call Corpco. Although the company's name has been changed to protect its anonymity and its employees' privacy, the overall picture of the corporate emotional health program is faithful to the facts revealed to me in interviews, case records, and field notes from January 1981 to November 1981. Corpco's program was an excellent setting for this research. It is considered a leader in the emotional health program movement, and its structure approximates the emerging behavioral medicine model discussed in earlier chapters.

The company

Corpco is located in the New York metropolitan area, and its EHP is nationally recognized for both its leadership and innovativeness. The company employs approximately six thousand people (43 percent male and 57 percent female). Managers are most often men, and lower-level employees are most often women. Currently, women compose 25 percent of management and 68 percent of lower-level employees. Corpco is not unionized and pursues a wide range of personnel policies designed to keep its work force nonunion (e.g., competitive salaries, excellent fringe benefits, flexible working hours).

The company agreed to participate in the research because the program director was deeply committed to research, believing that one sign of program maturity is the ability to examine one's own behavior and learn from that examination. He was confident that the research would provide useful information for future program development and thought that the research would enhance the program's image by demonstrating to employees that the company was doing something important enough to be studied. Finally, my hands-on experience made me a safe bet; it wasn't likely that I would disrupt the company's or the program's work.

Corpco is a company in transition. It is moving away from its paternalistic policies of the past (e.g., guaranteed employment) toward policies believed to be in line with "newer" marketplace realities. At the same time, it is trying to maintain the concern for employees reflected by its older policies.

Three years before the fieldwork, Corpco reorganized its

business structure and terminated many of its employees. This reorganization severely demoralized employees because it was in such sharp contrast to the old policies guaranteeing employment, and because employees had looked upon Corpco employment as a lifetime commitment. The shock of terminations stunned employees, and its reverberation could still be heard throughout the company even as a second reorganization was about to begin.

During the research period, Corpco, prompted by increasing competition in its markets, reorganized several of its operating divisions and terminated approximately three hundred fifty people. In order to economize, management cut budgets, reduced the number of employees, and introduced more sophisticated data processing equipment. Throughout the period, rumors of future cuts circulated among employees, for as Corpco inevitably moves toward increased computerization and automation, even more reorganizations and terminations can be expected. Indeed, Corpco's management predicts that in the not too distant future the entire company will be organized as a cottage industry in which employees will perform their jobs at video display terminals in their own homes.

The emotional health program

The EHP is part of Corpco's medical department, and its director reports to the corporate medical director. The medical department is large, consisting of five physicians and nine nurses (RNs and nurse practitioners), a wide variety of health services (e.g., annual physical exams, emergency care, occupational therapy), a well-stocked laboratory with the capacity to perform the latest medical tests, and a well-appointed library accessible to both the program staff and Corpco employees. Some staff members describe the department as equivalent to a small community hospital, and some question whether it is not too large and does not offer too many services to employees. Currently, the medical department is exploring the possibility of cutting some clinical services in order to economize. Those services that can be delivered more cheaply under the employees' insurance plan and through community resources may eventually be cut.

The evolution of Corpco's EHP closely parallels the history of other such programs over the last twenty-five years. In the 1950s, the medical department initiated it as an alcoholism program. During this period, the program consisted of a physician and an alcoholism counselor. In the early days, alcoholics were identified by their drinking behavior and referred to Alcoholics Anonymous; later, they were identified on the basis of deteriorating job performance and referred to residential alcoholism treatment programs as well. By the 1960s, the National Council on Alcoholism considered Corpco's program an outstanding example of what business could do for the employed alcoholic. Consequently, the physician became an activist in the alcoholism movement and promoted occupational programs. When public opinion focused on drug abuse in the late 1960s, the program expanded to include all substance abusers. When the employee assistance movement started in the early 1970s, the program expanded to include all "troubled" employees. At that time, a clinical psychologist, who eventually became program director, was hired to develop mental health services for employees. These services continue to make up the bulk of the program's offerings.

The program provides a number of services to employees and their families confidentially, free, and on company time. The staff use short-term cognitive-behavioral psychotherapy to treat employees. Generally, short-term psychotherapy consists of ten forty-five-minute sessions. Employees in need of longer term psychotherapy or highly specialized care are referred to an outside agency, institution, or practitioner covered under the company's mental health coverage. Also, employees concerned with confidentiality may ask to be referred to an outside practitioner. Alcoholics and drug abusers are referred to in-patient facilities for detoxification, intensive treatment, and ongoing follow-up. Staff members are on immediate call for crisis situations, such as suicide or homicide threats and psychotic episodes that might occur in the workplace.

Corpco's EHP is a pioneer in behavioral medicine. In the mid-1970s, the clinical psychologist began experimenting with biofeedback as a method for treating employees with stress-related illnesses. Using biofeedback and cognitive therapy, he taught employees to control such symptoms as headaches, backaches, and stomach problems and to manage stressors in their work and family lives. Biofeedback has become an important treatment technology in the program and is the basis for its stress-management training program. Because of its success, the EHP is searching for other behavioral approaches to apply to the prevention, diagnosis, and treatment of other physical and emotional problems. Planned prevention projects include stress reduction, alcoholism, obesity, and smoking.

As a general guideline the program maintains a staff of one therapist for every two thousand employees, but in times of stressful organizational changes this ratio has been increased to one therapist for every one thousand employees. During the study period the staff consisted of one full-time clinical psychologist, two part-time clinical psychologists, one part-time consulting psychiatrist, one full-time psychology intern (Ph.D. candidate), and two part-time psychology interns (M.A. candidates). By serving as a clinical psychology training site and by employing part-time clinicians, it is able to provide employees with a wide range of services at a reasonable cost to the company.

Although housed within the medical department, from January until May, the program was isolated from other medical department services in order to assure employees of maximum confidentiality. During May, however, the staff's offices were moved and integrated into the complex of consulting rooms used by the physicians and nurses for physical examinations and treatment. This move reflected the psychiatrist's medical orientation and his commitment to "holistic" medicine. He believed that the proximity of the psychologists to the physicians and nurses would encourage the medical staff to treat fewer patients with drugs and to refer them more frequently to the emotional health staff for behavioral treatment. My observations suggest that since the move, physicians and nurses have referred employees more frequently to the psychologists. Indeed, it is a more frequent sight to see a doctor or nurse leading an employee to the psychologists' offices in order to introduce them and arrange an appointment. The psychiatrist also claims to have seen a decrease in drug prescription.

Staying in Corpco

Once inside a field site, staying in requires developing rapport and trust with those being studied (Filstead 1970; Shaffir et al. 1980). From the beginning of the research, I sought to develop rapport and trust with all of the EHP staff members by informing them about the research and soliciting their help in talking with employees using the program. In two meetings, I met with them as a group and told them that I was interested in learning about the program and how employees chose to come there. At our first meeting, they listened politely and sought information about my background. They, however, remained skeptical about my interviewing employees because they feared a breach of confidentiality. During our second meeting, they agreed to invite employees to talk with me. They invited employees to speak with me at the end of the employees' first program visit. They asked employees to sign a release of information form as well. That form was developed in accordance with Corpco's and the federal government's guidelines on confidentiality, and it permitted me to interview the employees and review their EHP case records.

In the early days of my fieldwork, I visited the EHP on Tuesdays, Wednesdays, and Thursdays for at least a few hours each day. Between January and September 1, 1981, I spent 350 hours observing the program. Generally, I would stay in the EHP waiting area, where I would chat with the receptionist and observe and talk with employees as they came and went. The staff members were generally occupied either counseling employees or meeting about some program task (e.g., case reviews). These encounters were held behind closed doors and were accessible to me only in later discussions with the staff and employees. The longer I stayed and casually talked with the staff the more they seemed to accept me.

After several weeks, I noticed a shift in the staff's behavior toward me. They no longer seemed defensive about my talking with employees. Indeed, they seemed anxious to help me recruit them; and by late February I was beginning to interview a few of the program's clients.

Throughout the project, recruiting employees to interview was a frustrating task for the staff. They frequently apologized to me for not recruiting more, but employees' fears about confidentiality were a major barrier to their willingness to talk with me about their troubles. As one therapist explained, "I am sorry, Bill. I have got these guys who do not even want me to tell their own doctors that they are coming here. How can you expect them to participate?" And one employee commented to his therapist, "All medical records should be as confidential as possible. The fewer people with access to them the better." That included researchers.

By April, however, I was feeling fairly confident about my fieldwork. Interviews with employees were going slowly, but my relations with the staff were improving. Then the blow-ups occurred.

The clinical psychologist who had given me access was replaced by the psychiatrist who was not enthusiastic about my research project. This lack of enthusiasm stemmed, I believe, from his disagreements with the psychologist. The psychologist had been identified with the program for many years, and the psychiatrist had been with the program on a part-time basis for only a short time. Since the psychiatrist's arrival, they competed for control of the program. When the psychologist gave me entry, I unwittingly became identified as his ally, and with his promotion and departure, I was confronted with the necessity of working with the psychiatrist. He told me that I had allied myself with the wrong person, that he had questioned the project since my initial presentation, that the project would be canceled at the slightest hint of disrupting the program's work or relationship with management, and that he found it difficult to see how the staff could recruit any more employees because he and they had more important priorities.

It is fairly common for projects to be prematurely aborted because of changes in the company's personnel or political environment (e.g., Friedlander and Brown 1974). At such times, one learns that fieldwork entails continuous renegotiation of relationships (Shaffir et al. 1980). The EHP staff were very empathetic toward my situation and stated their continuing support of the project. They assured me that the psychiatrist was only trying to exert his control over the program, that I probably would not be thrown out, and that they would continue to help me. After all, as one of them confided to me, they too had experienced his tightening of the reins, and we were "all in this together."

My relationship with the psychiatrist did improve. Fortunately, before our meeting, I gave him a draft paper on the history of emotional health programs. Afterward, he read and made some helpful comments on it. The paper gave us something about which to talk constructively. From May until September, I saw very little of him because of his part-time schedule and summer vacation. However, when he was in the EHP, I always stopped by his office to say hello and ask how things were going. In his absence, I always tried to behave as a "welcome guest" (Wax 1980). At the end of my fieldwork, he graciously invited me to his private practice, where we spoke about the EHP for over three hours.

In June, there was a second blow to my fieldwork. At the time I had started the field research, the program was employing seven people full and part time, and by the end of June the staff was cut back to the part-time psychiatrist and one full-time therapist. Two staff members were clinical psychology students doing unpaid work at Corpco in order to satisfy their internship requirements. Upon completing their internships, they left the company. Reductions also occurred when the program's budget was cut, which necessitated terminating the two consulting psychologists.

The remaining therapist was also an intern and her tenure was due to expire in September. She was very empathetic toward my fieldwork because she too was completing a doctoral dissertation. Consequently, during the months of July and August, she made a great effort to keep me informed about the EHP and to help me talk with more employees. Due to increasing administrative demands on her time, however, she saw fewer employees and referred the majority of them to therapists outside of Corpco.

By September, my observations and discussions were recorded in over four hundred pages of field notes. I had interviewed thirty employees about their decision to use the EHP. When these conversations were tape recorded and transcribed, the transcripts ran to over fifteen hundred pages. In October and November, I turned to interviewing the EHP staff about their experiences.

Informants and respondents

Fieldwork yields data from many sources, including informants and respondents (Denzin 1978; Whyte 1979). Respondents are those individuals who simply respond to the researchers' questions. Informants take a more active role in the research, often becoming the eyes and ears of the researchers when they are not in the field to observe. Ideally, informants trust the investigator, freely give information about their problems and fears and frankly attempt to explain their

55

own motivations, demonstrate that they will not jeopardize the study, accept information given them by the researcher, and provide information and aid that could jeopardize their own careers.

In varying degrees, the EHP staff members acted as informants. As they came to trust me, they acted freer with me, often taking time to teach me about the EHP and its activities. In exchange for their good will, I advised them on their research proposals. Consequently, when I conducted my exit interviews with them in October and November, they were very forthright with me about their EHP experiences, confirming many of the insights from my field notes and illuminating some darker corners of the program.

The employees I interviewed were for the most part respondents. Corpco discouraged the staff from initiating contact with employees. For example, when employees broke an EHP appointment, staff members were not allowed to phone them because Corpco believed this would be perceived by employees as harassment. As a "welcome guest," I too was bound by this norm, which made it difficult to cultivate a closer relationship. However, I was able to keep in touch with a few employees I occasionally met in the medical offices, the hallways, or the cafeteria. Generally, they would inquire about my work and bring me up to date on their own cases. I listened, made mental notes, and recorded these insights in my field journal.

The thirty employees whom I interviewed were not a random sample. Indeed, confidentiality guidelines prevented the compilation of a list from which such a sample could be drawn. The employees were generally middle class and fairly well educated (most had at least one year of college). They comprised a wide spectrum of occupations from clerks to vice presidents and ranged in age from twenty to sixty-one years. Nineteen were women; eleven were men. All characterized themselves as coming to the EHP voluntarily (i.e., self-referred). As a whole, they are typical of the employees I observed coming and going in the EHP.

Interviews with employees ran from forty-five to sixty minutes and were scheduled to be compatible with the employee's work schedule. Most were scheduled and completed within a week of the employee's first visit to the EHP. Interview length was prescribed by an agreement with the program director to limit interviews to one clinical period. Corpco requested this to assure that work flow would not be seriously disrupted. Management-level employees usually requested to be interviewed in their offices. I gladly agreed to this request because it afforded access to parts of Corpco I would not ordinarily have seen. Interviews with lower echelon employees were conducted in a vacant medical office where privacy was assured.

In the interviews, I reassured employees that whatever they shared with me would be kept in confidence and that my writings would preserve their anonymity. The interviews were open-ended and focused on what employees knew about their problems and the EHP, how they acquired this knowledge, how they managed their problems, and why they decided to come to the program now. Throughout the interviews, I was concerned with maximizing the discovery process. To achieve this end, I followed up important leads as they emerged in the interviews.

Validity and reliability

Validity and reliability are issues for all research, and they concern the accuracy of the observations and concepts that researchers use to explain the phenomenon being studied. In survey research, reliability generally refers to a survey instrument's ability to accurately measure the same concept each time it is used, and validity generally refers to the capability of several different instruments to measure the same concept. Assurance of validity and reliability indicates that concept does exist in the group's behavior and is not merely the result of researchers' imaginations or testing biases.

In fieldwork, researchers use a variety of methods to study a particular phenomenon, but usually they rely upon participant observation, wherein the researchers are the instruments for measuring concepts. A reliable observation is one that is not biased by the idiosyncracies of the observer, a research instrument, a subject, or the constraints of time and place. It is an observation that could have been made by any similarly situated observer. The same, or nearly the same, behaviors would have been recorded in a field note or on any research instrument by any other observer. Observations that meet these criteria are considered reliable (Denzin 1978, 105). A valid observation is one that can be observed in the behavior of the group being studied. The researcher may observe the behavior directly or indirectly through informants or the analysis of documents. The more often the behavior occurs in the group and the more ways that it can be observed, the greater the validity of the observations.

In generating the description and theory about how employees decide to go to the EHP (chapter 4), I relied on employee interviews and field notes. The validity and reliability of these data are somewhat a problem. Those employees who agreed to be interviewed generally appeared to answer my questions honestly and to the best of their ability, and I believe that they would have been equally truthful about their experiences with other researchers. Consequently, this material probably adequately reflects their experiences in deciding to go to the program. I am uncertain, however, about the bias introduced by the employees' ability to select themselves for interviews. Other studies are needed to sort out this issue.

In developing the description and theory of EHP processes in chapter 5, I relied upon my field notes, employee case records, staff interviews, and psychotherapy literature reviews. I believe that this material accurately reflects how the staff processes employees who refer themselves to the program. Since I used my field notes to construct the staff interviews, I was able to compare many of the responses with the field notes. Where this was possible, there was a great deal of agreement. Generally, staff members appeared to answer my questions candidly and honestly. I believe this openness was a function of the rapport built up with them over months.

In sum, I believe that this report accurately depicts the manner in which employees choose to refer themselves to Corpco's EHP and the manner in which the EHP staff diagnose, refer, and treat employees.

Generalizability

Case studies raise questions about the extent to which findings can be generalized to other settings, and several characteristics of Corpco itself may limit the generalizability of the findings from this study. Corpco's EHP is firmly based within its medical department. Many companies do not have a medical department and locate their programs within personnel departments. Despite the medical concepts employed by the latter programs, the lack of physicians, nurses, and medical technology may cause the referral process there to be different. Also, Corpco's program serves as a training site for clinical psychologists; consequently, it is able to provide employees with a relatively large in-house counseling staff. Since most companies provide neither training to clinical psychologists nor a large in-house counseling staff to their employees, discretion should be used in generalizing these findings.

Overall, the theory from this study has fairly high generalizability because it is grounded in empirical observations. As researchers study other EHPs, they will inevitably modify and elaborate upon it. At present, however, practitioners can begin to apply the insights from this study to develop and evaluate their own programs.

4. Deciding to use the emotional health program

Before deciding to go to any treatment resource for help, people first must define their troubles as ones that require medical expertise and then choose a program that can help them. Usually, people learn that their troubles are medical ones when they seek and receive advice from their family and friends. In the process of seeking and receiving advice, they also learn about specific programs and how to use them. This chapter examines the process by which employees define their troubles as medical ones and decide to use Corpco's emotional health program.

Much of the research on defining emotional health problems emphasizes official labeling of trouble by social control agencies (e.g., police, mental hospitals). The initial identification and informal labeling of trouble has received less attention. Several studies on mental and physical illnesses, however, concur that it is not necessarily a change in behavior that causes trouble to be identified; it is, rather, a change in the significant audience. For example, Marian Yarrow and colleagues (1955) found that wives "normalize" their mentally ill husbands' behavior until third parties intervene. Peter Conrad (1976) found that parents and teachers normalize children's hyperactive behavior until it becomes a management problem, and Joel Telles and Mark Pollack's study (1981) of how individuals legitimate their physical illnesses suggests that the reactions of families, friends, and coworkers, rather than any actual change in their physical conditions, are instrumental in helping these individuals to decide that they are ill.

Since all the employees in my sample were being treated within the EHP at the time of this study, all of them were defined as having medical problems. This chapter is an exploratory analysis, based largely upon employees' self-reports, of the process of defining their concerns as medical problems. My conclusions, therefore, are tentative and suggestive rather than definitive.

The presenting problems

Employees who referred themselves to the EHP presented what they believed were appropriate problems for that resource: physiological, relational, and work-related problems. Physiological is the largest category of presenting problems, followed by relational and then work-related. The very large proportion of physiological problems that employees presented to the EHP suggests that they perceived the EHP as a medical program.

Twenty-four employees (80 percent) presented physiological problems to the EHP. The majority of these were stress-related. Employees reported generalized tension and nervousness; headaches; pains in the neck, lower back, chest, and jaw; stomach upset; elevated blood pressure; inability to sleep; tiredness; choking; and hyperventilation. Included as physiological problems were those of one employee who was upset about the removal of her uterus, one employee who referred himself for alcoholism treatment, and one employee who wished to quit smoking.

Four employees (13 percent) presented relational problems to the EHP. One employee reported difficulties with her parental family (e.g., curfews) and her boyfriend (Is he Mr. Right?). Three employees reported difficulties either with separation and divorce or with involvement with a new lover.

Two employees (7 percent) presented work-related problems to the EHP, one seeking career counseling and another seeking advice on how to handle a young M.B.A. who was increasingly taking over her assignment.

Seldom are problems so clearly delineated as these categories suggest. Although employees present one problem, they are usually concerned with other problems as well. When interviewed, employees who presented physiological problems were also experiencing relational problems, work problems, or both; and persons who presented problems with work or relationships reported feeling physiological distress.

Fifteen of the twenty-four employees who presented physiological problems (62 percent) associated those problems with their work. But the relationship between the physiological and the work problems was not always clear to the employees. Some reported the association and made no claims for causality, and some claimed that the physiological problems were directly affected, if not caused by, their work situations.

Jane W., thirty years old, came to the program seeking relief from what she described as a generalized tension and nervousness. She felt tense and nervous only when she was at work. She did not know what was causing her to feel this way but believed it was time to find out. She hoped the EHP could provide an answer.

Martin B., twenty-eight years old, came to the program with elevated blood pressure. He contended that his blood pressure was high only when he was at work. His mother, a registered nurse, regularly checked his blood pressure at home, and it was always within the normal range. But, when it was checked in Corpco's medical department, it was invariably high. Martin claimed his elevated blood pressure began when his department was reorganized last year. He described his new manager as a "screamer" who piled on the work while systematically undercutting his authority and organizational support. He particularly resented her "theory X management style" and the verbal abuse she gave employees.

Roy K., fifty-five years old, came to the program with blood pressure that he described as being "on the high side of normal." His mother was diabetic, and his father had died of a heart attack at an early age. Consequently, Roy felt he was susceptible to high blood pressure and monitored it frequently. Lately, the financial market had been fluctuating wildly, and the rumors about Corpco's reorganization had him a bit worried. His blood pressure appeared to fluctuate with the market and rumors.

Lorraine P., forty-nine years old, came to the program with complaints of sleeplessness and back pain. At first, she simply stated that most menopausal women had such complaints. Then she recounted that her promotion was in jeopardy because of conflicts with her new boss, a male, younger executive whom she had once managed and with whom she violently disagreed. After consideration, she estimated that 10 percent of her sleeplessness and back pain was due to menopause and 90 percent was due to her work situation.

The relationship among problems was even more complex for the eight employees who presented physiological problems that they associated with both their work and their personal relations.

Kevin D., fifty-one years old, came to the program with high blood pressure, which he traced to Corpco's previous reorganization and the near-death of his wife. Two years earlier, a very "stressful time" for Kevin, it had been touch and go whether he would be "out-placed,"[1] and it had been particularly difficult for him to stand by and watch some of his closest friends "forced out." During the same period, his wife had pneumonia and almost died.

Paul P., thirty-two years old, came to the program with

---

1. "Outplacement" is a euphemism for sending employees to a career counselor when the company fires them. During the reorganization, Corpco outplaced employees whose jobs were no longer considered essential. Typically, outplacement counseling consists of advising employees that their fears of not finding another job are irrational, assuring them that they need not worry about lost benefits (e.g., pensions), teaching them to write a resumé, and training them to find the "hidden job market." Outplacement agencies do not have listings of job openings and do not locate jobs for their clients.

migraine headaches. He described himself as a recreational marijuana smoker, and at first he attributed the headaches to smoking. Generally these headaches came and went quickly, but recently he had had one that lasted ten weeks. He did not know what had caused it, but feared organic damage. He also believed that the headache was probably due to his anxiety over his son's birth and his wife's quitting her job. He was worried about how he would support his family on his current salary and believed his present job was a dead end.

Patricia O., forty-one years old, came to the program with complaints of choking on food. She described her choking as a "bad habit," which had gotten worse that year. It embarrassed her, so she was eating lunch alone in her office. She felt that the choking episodes had become more frequent as both her work and family life became more troublesome. At home, she and her second husband were unable to talk to one another, and she increasingly found herself refereeing fights between her husband and children. At work, her boss was making unreasonable and conflicting demands because of his developing "alcoholism." After lunch, he was usually argumentative and found fault with everything she did.

Employees who presented relational and work-related problems to the program also experienced physiological distress.

Diana D., twenty-eight years old, came to the EHP feeling depressed about her separation from her husband and her relationship with her new lover. Having experienced an unhappy first marriage, she was uncertain whether she wanted to continue with the new relationship. She enjoyed being on her own and feared her personal and financial independence might be in jeopardy, because there was talk of reorganizing her department. She reported having a lot of headaches lately and breaking down and crying several times at work.

Mary M., thirty-five years old, came to the program with work problems. She had taken her present job because it offered both a challenge and an opportunity for advancement, but having conquered the assigned task, she suddenly found her advancement blocked by a young M.B.A. who took the credit for her work and systematically maneuvered her into a subservient role. Mary was angry, and taking that anger home was hurting her relationship with her boyfriend. She was "losing a lot of sleep," "very anxious and tense," and "very unhappy."

As the employee interviews made clear, the problem that an employee chooses to present for treatment is often one of several with which he or she is grappling. The physiological problems that employees present are usually caught up with turbulent work or family lives, and, conversely, the work or relational problems that employees present are caught up with physiological symptoms. The particular problem presented depends upon the process by which the employee reaches the EHP. In this process, the person forms ideas about what is an acceptable problem and its relationship to other problems.

The path by which employees travel to the EHP begins at a phase of containment, when employees are aware of their problems as discreditable attributes and attempt to manage signs, symptoms, and information about them in order to avoid being stigmatized. Employees particularly fear that, if their discreditable attributes become known to management, they will be evaluated harshly and possibly even fired. So they use several strategies to control information about their attributes and several tactics to contain the signs and symptoms. These tactics are directed primarily toward concealing the problems from management, but many of them work equally well in concealing problems from coworkers, friends, and family.

Several authors use the concept of containment. Steven Spitzer (1975) conceptualizes containment as the geographical segregation (e.g., prison) of troublemakers. Edwin Schur (1980) expands the term to include interpersonal, economic, visual, pharmacological, electronic, and physical forms of control. Angelo Alonzo (1979) uses the term to explain why some medical problems go unreported. He theorizes that illnesses go unreported because the individuals are able to contain the signs and symptoms of their conditions. Recognition of illness, then, occurs when there is a cumulative decline in an individual's ability to contain signs and symptoms and when such signs and symptoms disrupt social interaction at work, at home, or in the community. Following Alonzo's use of the term, I hypothesize that employees refer themselves to the EHP when containment breaks down and they are no longer able to control information about, and signs and symptoms of, their discreditable attributes.

Discreditable attributes

Any personal characteristic, behavior, condition, or quality carries the potential for being stigmatized (Schur 1979 and 1980). Employees revealed that a variety of personal characteristics that are not readily visible to others carry stigma potential. They recognize that if some act, quality, or characteristic of theirs were to become generally known, they might be stigmatized by their friends, coworkers, or employer. The problem, then, for an employee is to control information about the discreditable attribute (Goffman 1963). As Joseph Schneider and Peter Conrad (1980) illustrate, some people of necessity know about one's secret (e.g., family); rather, the employee's goal is to prevent that secret from being known by an ever-widening audience. While the employees' family members frequently are aware of their discreditable attributes, coworkers and supervisors usually are not aware, and most employees attempt to conceal this information from them.

Employees considered a wide range of attributes to carry stigma potential: being nervous, having attempted suicide, certain physiological conditions, a broken marriage, and a perceived decline in work performance.

Jane W., speaking about her nervousness and the consequences of its becoming known to management:

> I figured that if I did not get it taken care of now I would hurt myself. I would not get promoted. You know these

managers, they do not want someone who is nervous around them.

George M., speaking of his family, coworkers, and manager learning about his stress:

> The idea of stress and my projecting myself as not being the powerhouse, the nerves-of-steel guy [that] I think I project myself as being, would have been too shattering to me in terms of their image of me to reveal that. And to make them aware that you are not as strong as [they] thought you were, I think that would have been belittling to me. The reason is that I hold other people's opinions of me very highly, and as a result I destroy my image in their eyes.

Norton B., speaking about others finding out about the suicide attempt that precipitated his marital separation:

> I knew I had to tell him [the psychologist] about that [suicide attempt], and if this did go into the records—if anybody decides to look at these records and they see this kind of guy is working for us—well, that is the bottom line.

Beverly P., speaking of her embarrassment at having to explain temporomandibular joint syndrome (TMJ)[2] to others:

> They were all shocked. They said, "I never heard of such a thing." I never dreamed that a person's face could hurt. When I'm talking to people, they think that I am crazy. "How could it possibly hurt you? Your face? I could see your arm, your leg, but your face?" I said, "Yes, my face." It makes you feel stupid.

---

2. The joint between the upper and lower jaws is called the temporomandibular. Temporomandibular joint syndrome refers to pain and to problems in manipulating the jaw that are caused by spasms of the muscles associated with the joint. The pain is facial, often localized in the jaw or ear, and may extend down the neck to the shoulder. The person is unable to open his or her jaws fully and may suffer further limitations as well in jaw movement.

Ann Z., speaking about the loss of her uterus and its effect upon her prospects of finding a husband:

> Well, I guess I was convinced that I was never going to find a man in my life. People want families. Now there was no doubt. There was another strike, and that would be it.

Patricia O., speaking about the embarrassment caused by her choking on food when she eats in public, relating that several women teased her about her slow eating:

> I did not even want to sit in the cafeteria. I said I could see it was getting worse. There would be days when I just wanted to get up and run out of there.

Terri A., speaking about the shame she felt when her husband left her:

> I was too proud for my father, my aunts, and my uncles. I also felt at the time I was branded. I felt ashamed. I felt that I had failed. And 100 percent my fault. I did everything wrong. I was able to tell Angela and my sister, but I could not say that to my father.

How do employees learn certain of their attributes are discreditable? Howard Becker (1973) suggests that people recognize their own acts, qualities, and characteristics as being troublesome and are aware of certain relevant prohibitions in the larger cultural and social setting. This is particularly true of corporate cultures, which place a high value on conformity and self-control (e.g., Whyte 1957; Kanter 1977; Scott and Hart 1979). Indeed, in organizational America, the socialization process from cradle through school and into work teaches the employee to conform and to exercise self-control over his or her behavior, feelings, desires, and emotions in order to accomplish the organization's prescribed task. Again and again in the interviews, employees expressed a fear of losing control or of being seen by coworkers and managers as out of control. Those who expressed concern over feelings of nervousness and anxiety feared others would interpret these signs as indicating they were unreliable and might explode. Norton B. believed that his suicide attempt was the ultimate symbol of losing control—a belief reinforced by his sister's shocked expression when he tried to tell her about it.

Norton's experience also illustrates the second way in which employees learn they have discreditable attributes. They learn it when others react with such emotions as shock, surprise, and disgust. The employee feels ashamed and devalued, and such reactions can have an even greater impact upon employees who do not know of others with similar conditions. For example, neither Beverly nor Patricia knew anyone with TMJ or choking problems; nor did they know anyone who knew someone with these conditions. When others reacted negatively to their conditions, neither person had experience by which to gauge her own condition, and both felt isolated and wished to meet others with similar problems.

Joseph Schneider and Peter Conrad (1980) suggest a third manner in which individuals learn they have discreditable attributes. Significant others (e.g., parents and spouses) coach the individual on their vulnerability to stigmatism. While I have no direct evidence of such coaching in this sample, I suspect that in the cases of at least two women who were distraught about their ability to perform gender roles successfully, Ann Z. and Terri A., the women's relatives coached them on the necessity of concealing their conditions.

Controlling information

Usually employees learn to adopt strategies of concealment in order to control information about themselves. As George M. succinctly describes it,

> I have opened up too much, and I have found out it has
> hurt me. . . . The least they [management and coworkers]
> know about me personally the more it may benefit me,
> based on my experience.

Keeping quiet is one strategy used by employees to control information. It is straightforward and easily accomplished since many of the employees' problems are not readily observable by others. Marital problems, for example, are relatively easy to conceal from coworkers because work and family relations are usually separate. As long as the employees control the outward signs of emotional distress, they need not even discuss the matter. An example of a physiological problem that can easily be concealed is hypertension, which employees need not mention unless it becomes so troublesome as to either disrupt their performance or remove them from the workplace entirely. As one employee remarks,

> No, [I never discussed it.] Not with my family or with
> anyone else because I have really not had that much
> concern per se. I am aware of it, and I try to do certain
> things to lessen it.

Much the same can be said of the other stress-related physiological problems that employees present to the EHP. As long as the problem can be contained, there is no need to be too concerned, and it is relatively easy to conceal it from others.

It is also possible to conceal work-related problems from one's coworkers. Mary M.'s statement illustrates her movement from keeping quiet about her conflict with the M.B.A. to telling select coworkers about it:

> In the beginning, I was keeping it to myself because I
> felt it was not good to share these kinds of problems
> with coworkers. Because you never know what kind of
> reaction you will get. You never know who talks to whom.
> Since I notice that everyone else has the same grievance
> that I have, we discuss it.

Selective telling is another strategy to control information (Schneider and Conrad 1980). One generally tells trusted others, who are expected to keep one's confidence, about problems. The purpose of such telling seems twofold: to ascertain from the trusted other that one's problem is within some normal range and to obtain the trusted other's advice on managing the problem. As one woman states, "You do not do these things to find out that you have got something; you do them to see if you are all right."

Receiving helpful advice ("take it easy") from others appears to be an important factor in demonstrating that a problem is within the normal range and containable. Jane W. spoke with a coworker about feeling tense and nervous.

> I have a friend. . . . We work together, and I would mention it to her sometimes. "Mary, I don't know why I'm so nervous today." Like I said, it is not every day, but every day it is there somewhat. And not to the point where I am shaking a lot. . . . She just sort of said, "Go to bed; take it easy; try not to work too hard." Because I have got two kids. And stuff like that.

Another factor in helping to normalize the employee's concern appears to be some perceived standard of comparison. For Jane, the standard was "the point where I am shaking a lot." For George M., it was the opportunity to compare his stress reactions with those of his coworker and to conclude jointly that the symptoms were normal responses to their workload.

> I discussed it with my coworker, Bill. . . . The stress is getting to him too because at one point the both of us were getting headaches repeatedly. And we both thought that maybe the fact we always have this door closed, some poisonous gas or something was coming in here through the ventilation system. We found that we were only getting the headaches in this room. So as it turns out, I do not believe that there is any kind of toxic fumes

being pumped in here through the ventilation system. It is more the fact that we confine ourselves in here like we are in prison. Pumping out the work. We want to get things done. While everyone outside is talking about baseball and football, we are in here with our nose to the grindstone.

In instrumental telling, a form of selective telling (Schneider and Conrad 1980), employees seek to disavow or deny others' comments or perceptions of them and to give what they believe is a more acceptable account of themselves. For example, Patricia O. finally told "the girls" about her choking in order to avoid their teasing and to demonstrate that her behavior was rational:

> I was getting teased by those who did not know. I eat lunch on occasion with girls who work in the department. I usually eat exclusively with one girl, and when she is not in, I eat with the others. And they would tease me about it. So I finally did tell them about it. And they felt bad. I did not want to advertise what it was.

By revealing her choking response, Patricia was able to elicit a more sympathetic reaction from her coworkers.

Norton B. told his boss and coworkers about his marital separation, but not about his attempted suicide, when he feared that the emotional distress from "it all" was beginning to affect his job:

> I did ask my boss that [whether my marital problem was affecting my performance]. And I asked my supervisor and a couple of people at work that I associate with. I asked them because I really could not tell. The type person that I was and when I was going through this, which was actually around the holiday time, they could tell that something was bothering me—"He was not his cheerful self." I was just low key. So I knew I was visible. No. I inquired, and the answer that I got back was "no" that it did not interfere with my work at all.

In addition to statements that his performance was satisfactory, Norton's account also elicited sympathy and assurances that his behavior was normal and containable.

Network building is an important form of selective telling. It is the primary way in which employees seek to handle work-related problems. They discuss their problems with select other employees in order to obtain either a transfer out of their department and into another or advice on how to handle problems created by their current job. Usually, they prefer obtaining the transfer to receiving advice. Such discussions are usually held with those higher-level managers with whom an employee has developed some rapport or friendship. Frequently, these managers were once either the employee's co-worker or supervisor, and the employee has reason to believe that the manager will be sympathetic.

Lorraine P. spoke to a dozen people about finding an alternative position within Corpco. Her search was more extensive than those of most other employees, which reflected both her long tenure (twenty-six years at Corpco) and her popularity with others. The senior and middle-level managers with whom she spoke all agreed that her previous boss had been derelict in not promoting her to assistant vice president and agreed to help her in developing a transfer. Indeed, her search was in progress when I arrived for our interview. She was talking with someone on the phone. When I inquired about the conversation, she replied,

> That was one of the friends that I had talked to, and he had sent me to somebody else. Hopefully, it would open some doors. "Maybe I could get a transfer?" You heard me say that. And that man said, "If you can go to another [job] area, go. With regionalization there are so many people that are being out-placed that any other openings will be taken. But people are in far more desperate situations than you are."

Network building can become a run against the clock. Will the employee find a transfer before the current work situation breaks down and results in a major confrontation with the boss? To cope with this contingency, employees tend to set deadlines for finding a transfer and beginning a job search outside the company. Lorraine had set July 4 as her deadline, although she admitted having previously established May 31 as the deadline. As July 4 drew near and her prospects for a transfer looked brighter, she was beginning to think that perhaps she would decide later in the summer, after her vacation.

Given the difficulties in obtaining transfers, sometimes the only thing others can do is advise the employee on how to handle the work problem more effectively. Mary M. had such a discussion with an older woman executive.

> When I was going to talk to my boss, she sort of advised me on how to approach him [Mary's boss]. She told me, "Don't be negative. Don't go there feeling emotional; come down first and think what you are going to say. Always put it in the positive side. Don't accuse him of anything. Just ask questions. And even rehearse if you have to." Yeah! She was very, very helpful. The first time that I talked to her we had lunch and sort of rehearsed it.

Elizabeth T. partially attributed her headaches to the many work demands made upon her. A former coworker counseled her to slow down and be more realistic about what could and could not be accomplished.

> I think he was one of the first people to point things out to me and say, "I can't believe it. I mean this does not have to be done in an hour. And you've got the wrong concept. This is not the most important thing in the world." . . . And then I realized. Boy, it is silly. It is not the beginning and end of life here. So between a little bit of him and my ears and a little bit of my own realization that there is something to this, I have been able to help myself a little bit.

Not everyone is nearly so successful as Lorraine, Mary, and Elizabeth. When I interviewed Salvatore I., his time was running out. His discussions with others had not produced either hope of a transfer or helpful advice; consequently, he had already begun to look to his "buddies" outside of Corpco for another job and had begun to feel the despair employees experience when networks break down.

> See, I talked to one of the fellows who is a V.P. . . . And I knew him for years before that. He used to tell me what to do, and he told me, "Just give it time. Don't get depressed. Just give it time. I know it is hard on the job. It is hard work, but you have to give it time." Then I talked to someone else, and they said the same thing, "You've got to give it time." I said, "You can only give it time, so much time, and then you run out of time."

Network building gives employees a sense of getting the work problem under control, and it also helps to normalize their experiences. Through selective conversations, employees learn that their work experiences may be unpleasant and their bodies may react in uncomfortable ways but that such conflict, competition, and unpleasantness is a "normal" part of corporate life.

Tactics for managing signs and symptoms

In addition to controlling information about their discreditable attributes, employees also use several tactics to manage directly the signs and symptoms of their problems: ingestion of chemicals, relaxation techniques, professional consultation, and workplace tactics.

Chemical ingestion, including such activities as dieting, drinking alcohol, smoking marijuana, vitamin therapy, and using prescribed and over-the-counter medication, is employed to control the physical and psychological distress that employees experience. Employees learn to use these methods from previous experiences with physicians, friends, and relatives and from reading magazine and newspaper articles.

Diet was a popular strategy for containing signs and symptoms of headaches and high blood pressure. Dieters reported that they and their family members were alert to new diet articles and tried to use the ideas presented. Migraine sufferers would often try to trace the onset of a headache to something they ate, and they claimed that dairy products, chocolate, and caffeine produce headaches.

Closely allied with diet is vitamin therapy. One woman reported using B_6, B_{12}, and kelp to prevent headaches, a technique learned from articles given to her by her mother. She stated that her headaches seemed less severe and less frequent since she started using vitamins and that their onset occurred when she ran out of any one of the vitamins.

Males reported using alcohol and marijuana to cope with stress. United States culture supports alcohol use as a means of unwinding (e.g., Bacon 1962), and employee interviews confirmed that attitude. They generally reported drinking with others in restaurants, social clubs, and bars. Each reported that at one time he had feared reliance on alcohol was turning him into an alcoholic. For all but one of the males, this worry was alleviated when they found they could stop drinking for extended periods of time. The one marijuana smoker reported using marijuana in a similar manner, and at one time he too feared becoming addicted.

Employees reported mixed feelings about using prescribed and over-the-counter drugs to contain signs and symptoms. Most expressed displeasure at using prescription drugs and preferred to use Tylenol or the "odd aspirin." Even the use of aspirin, however, was not always whole-heartedly condoned, because, as one woman stated, "For every aspirin you take, you lose a drop of blood from your heart." The displeasure at using drugs was usually founded on some previous unpleasant experience with a physician's prescription. Again and again, respondents reported that some drug had incapacitated them, had made them feel like zombies, and had interfered with their role responsibilities.

Elizabeth T.'s experience with prescribed medication for her headaches was fairly typical of the employees' complaints about prescription drugs.

I never tried to get anything. You know, maximum-strength Anacin is my best. I do not take to drugs too well. I think I have low tolerance. Dr. Gill had given me an antidepressant, which I took for 2 or 3 days and got a rash. So I stopped that and he gave me another one that also had a tranquilizer in it. I was reluctant about taking it. He assured me that it was very mild. I took the second one, and I went outside in the back to read. As soon as I got out there I said, "You are going to be in trouble if you do not get back into the house soon." I went back into the house, and I just collapsed on the living room floor. The next thing I remembered was the kids coming in from school. I mumbled something to them about, "Mommy is not feeling too well. I am just going to lie here." Then I went out again. A friend called; I got to the phone, but I could not speak well. So I thought that is it for that pill. So I really do not look for prescriptions.

Although watching what foods one eats, taking vitamins, drinking alcohol, smoking marijuana, and using some prescription and over-the-counter drugs can all help contain signs and symptoms, imprudent dosages of alcohol, marijuana, and other drugs create their own containment problems if they interfere with an individual's role requirements and engender adverse reactions from family, friends, and coworkers.

Relaxation techniques include prayer, meditation, self-hypnosis, and exercise. These techniques are used by both men and women for a wide range of stress-related problems (e.g., high blood pressure, backaches, generalized tension, and nervousness). Again, these techniques are learned from previous experiences with physicians, from family and friends, and from reading popular publications such as *The Relaxation*

Response (Benson 1975). Employees describe them as being fairly effective in helping to contain signs and symptoms. One executive who uses transcendental meditation and self-hypnosis to control his blood pressure stated that he had become so relaxed that he often forgets to practice the technique. An executive woman encouraged by a physician to exercise in order to reduce menopausal tension reported that the technique was working until her job blew up. With that additional strain, no amount of exercise really helped.

For many employees, the visit to the EHP was not the first time they had consulted a professional about their problems. Employees reported professional consultation with a family physician, specialist, helping organization, priest, or marriage counselor to help contain their problems. It is not always clear why the employee went to the particular professional at the time, but I suggest that the person went because the containment process broke down and they were encouraged to do so by family and friends. Having obtained the professional advice and regained control of his or her symptoms and signs, the employee integrated the professional advice into his or her repertoire of control techniques. Mary Margaret O.'s story illustrates this use of professional consults. She was twenty-nine and had had migraines off and on since she was fourteen. Over the years, usually at the instigation of her mother, she visited a number of professionals and organizations: her family physician, a neurologist, an opthamologist, and the Mt. Sinai Headache Clinic. When she was twenty, the eye specialist prescribed a tranquilizer for the headaches.

> I even went to an eye doctor, and he said they were migraines. He would just give me a prescription and say, "When you know you are getting the warning signs, take one and maybe you won't get them so bad." So for all these years, I have been going and getting my prescription refilled.

Another form of professional consultation reported by employees diagnosed as having high blood pressure and by those concerned about developing it was the use of Corpco's hypertension clinic to monitor blood pressure. This monitoring was generally combined with diet and relaxation techniques.

Not all professional advice is so helpful, and, consequently, not all professional advice is integrated into the employee's containment repertoire. Elizabeth T., for example, consulted a priest about her marital difficulties and found his advice "not particularly helpful."

Employees used a number of tactics—cover up, taking time out, and losing oneself in work—to contain signs and symptoms while at work and to handle work-related problems. To contain powerful emotions, employees typically cover up by temporarily removing themselves from their office or work station. Lorraine P.'s comments give insight into the meaning employees attach to crying:

> It is funny. I have an idea of emotional [illness] as somebody who is standing around crying in the halls. I have friends, people who I know really well enough to know if they have cried on their jobs; they all have. Without exception. A lot of people, I do not know if they have cried on their job, and I cannot imagine it. But when you know that 100 percent of the people that you know well enough to know whether they did or not have either gone into the ladies' room or gone into someone else's [office] (when they get up high enough, they do not dare go into the ladies' room for fear that someone else will come by and see them crying, so they have to go to a friend's office so they can cry), you realize that this does not mean they have gone off the deep end, but you have that idea of mental illness. . . . I think crying is ok if you hold on until you get to the bedroom and close the door. But it should never overtake you anyplace else.

In the United States crying is typically associated with women, and almost all the women interviewed mentioned being overcome with tears at some time. U.S. culture supports, or at least tolerates, such behavior in women, so it is not at all surprising that they admit to it.

The men interviewed did not admit to crying, but their descriptions of the powerful emotions they attempt to cover up make one wonder if they were close to tears. Norton B. told of covering up his emotions whenever he thought about being separated from his children:

> I thought about it. Like I am sitting at the table and all of a sudden I look up and see the kids, and I start getting emotional. Maybe I should disappear off the floor and get out? I said, "that ain't gonna do no good." I just kept my steady pace. Yes, there were times when I was waiting for work to be done and it clicked into my mind. Then, what I would do is get up and walk down the hall and shoot the breeze with somebody for a few minutes and come back and it was gone. I would go back to it again.

George M. spoke of covering up the symptoms of his nervousness:

> When I feel it coming on myself—my head getting cloudy and hyperventilating or getting hot flashes . . . I find a quick opportunity or excuse to escape from the situation. Go off and wash my face or walk and come back. I am reshaped again back to normal. Then I can deal with it.

Frequently, a quick trip to the restroom or a walk around the building does not provide sufficient time for the employee to regain control of his or her emotions and behavior. When this happens, employees opt for taking some time off, usually a half day from their vacation. While this tactic has the advantage of removing them from the sight of management and coworkers, it also has the disadvantage of keeping them away from work. Taking time off can lead to its own problems and become risky. Terri A. told of taking time off and explaining the reason to her coworkers:

As far as crying was concerned, if I saw myself doing that during the day, I would just leave. So, the area knew something was going on, but it was not until two months after [my husband] left that I actually had the courage to say even that my husband left.

Some employees lost themselves in their work and thereby banished their problems from their consciousness. For these individuals, work becomes time away from their problems. Ann Z. spoke of losing herself in work in order to forget the loss of her uterus. In addition to working at Corpco, she was a sales clerk and occasionally did paralegal work.

I work hard here. I really lost myself in work. And I have a second job that I started back when I first worked here. So I kept myself very busy, and I did not have much time. Two jobs and I did not have time to think about anything else.

Engrossment can and does break down, allowing the banished thoughts to flood the employee's consciousness. On such occasions, one's coworkers or supervisor may even suggest taking time off. Rita N. lost herself in work in order to forget her father's death, her cousin's murder, and her feud with her sister.

I managed to get through the day. I did not see any point in sitting home and dwelling on it. It did not do any good. So I forced myself to come to work. The more I did the less I thought about it. But I got upset a few times. My boss wanted to send me home, but I told him, "No, that is not necessary."

Reactions of others

The reactions of others to a particular behavior is a key variable. These reactions help individuals to formulate their feelings, attitudes, and actions toward the attribute in question

(Schur 1979). Because the research setting did not permit me to interview those close to the employees in the sample to obtain insight into their reactions toward the referred employees' behavior during the containment phase, the following remarks are based on the employees' statements and their perceptions of how others reacted to them.

Generally, all the employees reported a high degree of tolerance of their problems. In fact, several reported that others were more generous in their tolerance toward them than they would have been if the tables had been turned. Family and close friends were perceived as only slightly more tolerant than managers and coworkers. Although several women reported having to conceal their choking, headaches, and TMJ pain from their husbands, who were beginning to lose patience, and two men reported that their wives and children objected to their drinking, such negative reactions from families were the exception rather than the rule.

Why so much tolerance? The data suggest several reasons. First, employees were fairly successful in concealing their problems. Even though the employees were aware of their problems, coworkers and managers probably were not aware of the employees' problems. Second, when containment did break down, employees' proffered accounts appeared to be accepted—after all, everyone has a bad day. Third, the employees probably did not exceed the tolerance quotient built into work and family situations, and, if they did exceed it, the reactions of others were perceived by the employees as comparatively mild.

Coworkers appeared to accommodate themselves to the employee's bad days, which are perceived as being within normal limits, and the employee, through selective conversations, learns that his or her attribute, behavior, or condition is within normal limits and containable. If coworkers react with tolerance, accommodation, and normalization during the containment stage, how then does containment break down and the employee's behavior, condition, or attribute become defined as a medical problem?

Referral triggers: symptoms

Operationally, an employee's problem is defined as a medical problem when the employee decides to refer himself or herself to the medical or emotional health programs for either an examination or treatment. This de facto definition is really prelabeling, since only a medical professional can attach a medical label to the individual's problem, and should be differentiated from official labeling by medical professionals.

Several hypotheses about how containment breaks down and employees decide to seek help can be formulated. The most popular explanation among health care providers is simply that the symptoms become so serious and the discomfort from them so overwhelming that employees are compelled to come for treatment. This assumption underlies the studies of patient delays that characterize delay in seeking treatment as irrational (e.g., Fries and Ginsberg 1979).

James Greenley and David Mechanic (1976), studying students' decisions to use a university's counseling center, found that distress does have a direct effect upon the decision to refer oneself. My research at Corpco corroborates this, particularly in those cases where symptoms present themselves in a striking fashion.

Terri A. had known for months that her marriage was in deep trouble. She urged her husband to go to a marriage counselor, but he steadfastly refused. One evening he packed his bags, told her he was getting a divorce, and left. Terri was devastated, and the pain was overwhelming.

> I went berserk. I just wanted to kill myself. I did not just say that. I was actually thinking of ways to do it. I was not sleeping; I was not eating. . . . My heart was ripped out; my guts had been ripped out of me.

The following day, Terri referred herself to the EHP.

Beverly P. remembers the onset of her TMJ syndrome as sudden and painful. Within a few days, she set up an appointment with her dentist. The dentist misdiagnosed the pain and recommended several root canals, a process that added to Beverly's pain. When the pain did not subside, she went to a local emergency room where an intern diagnosed her problem as TMJ syndrome and referred her to a specialist who seemed unable to relieve her pain. After a series of consultations, she eventually ended up in Corpco's medical library.

> My jaws like lock. It has been like that for months. It is very painful, and I have not been able to find a doctor who can tell me that there is a cure for it. . . . It is just aggravating me and growing. So I said maybe if I go to the library and find out, do some research and find out what actually can be done about it. I read in several articles that a lot of people get frustrated because they cannot open their mouth.

When the librarian saw the articles that Beverly had been reading, she informed her about the EHP and its capacity to use biofeedback and relaxation techniques to reduce the TMJ syndrome. Beverly immediately left the library and set up an intake appointment with the receptionist.

While these cases illustrate the dramatic impact of symptoms on seeking help, symptoms alone do not and can not account for Terri's and Beverly's behavior. Equally important to Terri was the perception that, having lost her husband, she was a failure in her family's eyes. Equally important to Beverly was the perception that the TMJ pain made her less attractive to her husband, disrupted her social life, and interfered with her career. Even in those dramatic cases where pain seems greatest, social factors shape the referral process.

Typically, employees in the sample did not seek aid when they experienced the most physical discomfort. This was true whether the symptoms were for choking, migraine, hyperventilation, or generalized tension and nervousness. All experienced worse symptoms at other times, even those employees who reported that their symptoms were caused or exacerbated by work or family problems. According to my data, employees went to the EHP either when containment broke down or when the employee perceived that it was about to break down.

Referral triggers: cultural

The works of Marian Yarrow et al. (1955) and Irving Zola (1973) suggest that individuals seek help from psychiatrists and physicians not because of the symptoms per se but because of the meanings that the individuals learn to attach to these symptoms (Yarrow et al. 1955, Zola 1973). Zola found that patients who referred themselves to either the eye clinic, the ear, nose and throat clinic, or the medical clinic did not seek aid at their physically sickest point. Their decisions to seek medical aid were based on breaks in the individuals' accommodations to the symptoms. These breaks were precipitated by several distinct nonphysiological triggers: occurrence of an interpersonal crisis, perceived interference with social or personal relations, sanctioning, perceived interference with vocational or physical activity, and temporalizing of symptomology. While these decision-making patterns were used by all ethnic groups in Zola's sample, the triggers tended to cluster according to ethnicity, with Italians, Irish, and Anglo-Saxons using particular ones.

With the exception of temporalizing of symptomology, Zola's cultural triggers appeared to have precipitated employee referral to the EHP. Because of my small sample size, however, the relationship between triggers and ethnic groups in this sample was highly tentative. What is more conclusive, however, is that all groups reported these triggers as their reasons for seeking help. Employees appear to learn from their cultural and social settings the appropriate rationales for self-referral.

When interpersonal crisis prompted self-referral, the crisis called attention to preexisting symptoms and caused the patient to dwell upon them and finally to do something about them. The preexisting symptoms, then, provide the individual

85

a method of escaping from the interpersonal crisis. What breaks down is the individual's accommodation to the interpersonal crisis and not to the symptoms per se. Regardless of the reality and seriousness of the symptoms, they provide but the rationale and escape to a potential source of help.

Adelle D. was sixty years old and had worked for Corpco for eight years. Before working for Corpco, she was employed by a brewery company. When the brewery company closed its New York plant and moved to the South, she was distraught because her coworkers "were like family and everyone was so pleasant and helpful." About the time of the brewery's relocation and her move to Corpco, she started to have migraine headaches. She never felt close to her Corpco coworkers, and she believed that her hard work was unappreciated. She controlled her migraines with a mild tranquilizer and diet. When she had a headache at work, she went to one of Corpco's physicians, whom she described as "very understanding." So why did she go to the EHP?

> Last week was a horrible week. So much work and no one appreciated it. Despite my headache, I worked harder than anyone else. My supervisor prefers his own kind [he is black]. It is not like when I was at the brewery company. I tried to talk to him, but he does not care. He said, "If your headache is so bad, why don't you go to Medical?" So I did. Dr. Whyte sent me here.

Adelle was in the EHP for several months before being referred to a neighborhood mental health center for further help. Just before I finished data collection, Adelle came again to the EHP in tears, complaining about a headache and about her supervisor's and coworkers' lack of appreciation. When I asked a staff psychologist about Adelle, she replied, "Her. She is just a complainer. She thinks no one appreciates her. I told her to go home for the afternoon." Adelle used her headaches to escape, at least temporarily, once more.

The second triggering pattern, perceived interference with social or personal relations, is illustrated by Jeanette T. She had had a stressful year. Her father died after a long hospitalization; her mother suffered a cerebral hemorrhage; and Jeanette worked a series of sixteen-hour days. Throughout these experiences, she felt tired and exhausted, but despite these symptoms managed to cope. Just when things were beginning to return to normal, some additional work problems materialized, which required Jeanette to spend even more time away from family and friends:

> I did some traveling [and] work here. I thrive on that. I really, really thrive. So I cannot say it is just the hours. But you go home and you have like 2 hours for yourself. I enjoy my social life, and I had to give up some of that. Anyhow, I was feeling very, very tired. I think my blood pressure went up. I went and made an appointment with Dr. Rose.

Jeanette's blood pressure was normal. She did feel tired, but this was not the first time that she had felt so tired. What changed and triggered her decision to refer herself was the perception that the work demands and the subsequent tiredness were interfering with her personal and social relationships. It was the final straw.

The cultural trigger sanctioning consists of one person taking the primary responsibility for the decision to seek aid for someone else. Patricia O.'s choking had occurred on and off for fifteen years. She reported that it had increased of late because of her marital and work problems. Seeking relief from her marital difficulties, she encouraged her husband to accompany her to a psychologist for family counseling. After several sessions, during which Patricia's husband was uncooperative, the psychologist turned her attention to Patricia's choking and recommended either biofeedback or transcendental meditation as a possible cure. Within a few days, Patricia set up an appointment with the EHP.

> She said, "Why shouldn't you do something about it?" And I said, "That is what I have been thinking." [During]

the conversation [it came up] that it was time I did do something positive.

When asked why she had not done something about it before, Patricia replied that nobody had told her to do something before.

Sanctioning, however, does not always function alone. In some instances, someone may take the responsibility for the employee of making the decision to seek help, and the employee may choose to get further sanctioning from the employee network.

Maureen Mc. was twenty-one and lived with her father, stepmother, and three sisters. Her current boyfriend wanted to marry her, but she was not sure whether she was ready. She feared that she would become an alcoholic and die an early death like her mother. She was acting out by drinking and keeping late hours. Her family was concerned, and her stepmother had taken the responsibility of encouraging Maureen to come to the EHP. Maureen's stepmother knew of the program because her own sister, a Corpco employee, had used it with success.

> My mother said, "Maureen, would you like to talk to somebody?" Not "I think you should" or "I want you to," but "Would you like to?" That made me feel a lot better about it because she gave me the choice. . . . If they say do this, I am not going to do it. When they say would you like to and I know they would like me to do it, I will do it.

Maureen followed up her stepmother's urging with a conversation with a woman in her department.

> Then, I sit behind this girl, and I asked her a question, "Do they have anybody here to whom you can talk to about your problems?" She said, "Oh, yes!" . . . She said that she went, came down here when she really had a lot of problems. You know, with the person she was

living with. She said they helped her tremendously. So I thought maybe they could help me too.

The trigger, perceived interference with work or physical functions, occurred when employees perceived that their condition was about to interfere with their work. This is the one decision-making pattern that most closely approximates the EHP's raison d'être.

When I asked Jane W. why she came to the EHP now, she replied,

> Oh, I have had this problem for a while. I keep like putting it off. There are days when I am ok. What really made me decide to do something about it was that I got a promotion to a secretary for a V.P. I said I cannot go being all tense all the time and nervous. I have to be a little bit more stable. That is when I said maybe it is my blood pressure or something like that. So I had better have a physical done. That is when I explained it to Dr. Rose.

Shortly after Irene C. was nominated for an assistant vice presidency, she referred herself to the EHP for preventive assistance in coping with generalized stress, a condition she claims to have experienced "all of my life."

> I was not particularly involved with anything that was bothering me. It was more a general feeling of wanting to do the best you can. I was thinking about the future and the fact that my mother died of arteriosclerosis of the brain. I did not feel like going that route.

For some employees the perceived interference with work may not be sufficient motivation to refer oneself to the EHP. In George M.'s case, another employee familiar with the program provided additional impetus to the referral decision. George had had stress-related symptoms for several years. In fact, two years earlier, during a medical examination, a physician recommended biofeedback to him, and George refused. So why seek that treatment now?

It affected my work; it has also affected my personal life. When I am in a situation of stress, I feel stressful and all pent up. It is a time when I want to be left alone. . . . Like with my wife. I do not tell her, "Leave me alone now." I just let her say what she has to [say], and, then, I get so annoyed that I actually jump at her. Similarly at work, I jump at my coworkers sometimes. . . . I [also] had occasion last week to speak to one of my coworkers, and he mentioned that he was having similar stress-related problems and that he was trying to deal with them too. He mentioned that he had gone to biofeedback. . . . I decided, Jesus, maybe it is a good thing that I should get involved in that also. Because him and I had a discussion on that if I did not do something soon, I could end up getting sick. . . . I should mention one thing to you. [The coworker] may have been the kick in the ass, but I had it on the agenda, as a matter of fact, my little book, for the past couple months.

The day after his conversation with the coworker, George called the EHP for an appointment.

Referral triggers: workplace

While my data suggest that Zola's cultural triggers play an important role in breaking down containment, they also suggest that several structural characteristics of the workplace are influential: employee networks, supervisory discussions, and medical routines.

Typically, the employee network functions as a reaffirmation of the employee's decision to seek help and as a source of information about the EHP. The interaction between the employee and network member is characterized as a peer relationship, with the employee initiating conversation about his or her own problem. Such conversation usually follows rather than precedes the network member's revelation that he or she has used or is using the EHP with some success. In this sample, no network member gave the employee unsolicited advice about his or her problem. This is not to suggest that network members never give unsolicited advice, but it does suggest that coworkers respond to employees' specific inquiries. The employee network functions to inform the employee of the EHP's existence and to assure him or her of its efficacy.

Discussions between supervisors and employees are not conversations between peers. Even when employees report a close relationship with their supervisors, they recognize the supervisor's superior position and their own responsibility to maintain an appropriate level of performance. As one employee stated about her close relationship to her "very understanding" supervisor, "He just realizes there is a boundary, and he should not have to put up with that."

The quality of supervisory discussions varies tremendously, from the passing informal conversation to planned discussions bordering on formal performance appraisal. Interestingly, the passing informal conversations were associated with female employees, and the more planned, formal discussions were associated with male employees. In part, this reflects the circumstances surrounding the supervisors' interventions.

Ann Z., for instance, was struggling to contain her feelings about the loss of her uterus by losing herself in her work. One afternoon while at lunch she felt close to tears, and her luncheon companion urged her to take the afternoon off and go home. Ann refused, went back to her office, and was soon in tears. She phoned her boss's secretary to say that she was going home. Shortly after that, her boss came into her office, and as Ann relates,

> Everything was just coming down on my head, and I just started to cry. I do not remember everything. I guess the final thing was the problems and tension. I had tensed up and finally broke. I spoke to my boss. I could not have

91

> found a more sympathetic ear to talk to. He sat and
> talked with me for a while. Just to get things off my
> chest. Which helped. He recommended that, if I wanted
> to talk to someone down here, [I should call].

That afternoon Ann phoned to make an appointment. She
was unable to get an immediate one, and her boss checked
with her daily until she was able to do so.

Crying indicates to supervisors and managers that something is amiss and provides them with an excuse to intervene.
In fact, those managers included in the employee interviews
recounted similar interventions with distraught women as in
the case of Diana D.

> My boss suggested it to me because she knows basically
> that I am separated and that I am in the process of a
> divorce and that sometimes things are getting to me. . . .
> Well, that particular day I kind of broke down in the
> office and started crying. . . . That had happened a couple
> of times. That is when she saw the condition that I was
> in. That is why the suggestion was made.

Diana was unable to contain her distress, and apparently
her supervisor was unable to continue to accommodate her
tears. The situation with two of the males is somewhat different. Both were long-term employees, with eighteen and
thirty-two years of service, respectively. Both were encouraged by their supervisors to refer themselves for alcohol-related
problems. In both cases, a great deal of accommodation preceded the final supervisory intervention. What precipitated
these supervisory discussions and employee referrals? In the
first case, the employee, Salvatore I., acquired a new supervisor, whose job required her to whip the service agency into
shape. Where Salvatore's previous boss could tolerate him,
his new one probably could not. According to him, she in-
stigated the referral:

> What happened was my boss, she started in June of
> 1980. . . . She called me into her office and told me about

> my work production being low. I told her my attitude about the job. I did not hold anything back from her. I really did not know her that well. I told her I was doing the same job year in and year out, and after awhile it just gets to you. Well, she suggested that she felt I was spending too much time in the bar, which I used to do three or four times a week. . . . So, a couple of times, apparently, I came back from lunch and smelt a little of alcohol on my breath. She brought that up. I said that I do not think it is this. She suggested that I go for an examination. She set up an appointment with Dr. Greene.

This supervisory discussion bordered on a formal performance appraisal, and Salvatore complied with the supervisor's wish only after "looking up in the book" and finding that she could refer him to the medical department. He believed he could have refused, but decided to see the doctor because it might help with his job search.

The new manager forced Salvatore to refer himself by indirectly threatening his job. The second alcohol case also demonstrates how the threat of possible job action can stimulate referrals. Indeed, Dennis M.'s case is almost a classic statement of job threat as an inducement to enter alcoholism treatment. Dennis had been employed in his present job for over thirty years, and he reported having drunk heavily since he was sixteen. For the previous five years he had been very concerned about his drinking. Despite his wife's and daughter's prodding him to "quit," he had continued to drink and to avoid becoming involved with either AA or an alcoholism treatment program. Then while preparing for a fellow employee's retirement party, Dennis became drunk, and his boss sent him home to sleep it off.

> That is what really did it. . . . My manager saying [it] to me. . . . I left, but naturally I did not go right home. I went right across the street to [a bar] and had a couple of more drinks there. Then I stopped around the neighborhood. . . . When I was in my neighborhood, I started to

93

realize I more or less got kicked out of my job. But he did not fire me. He just suggested that I go home because of my condition. I said I better do something about this now. Besides, the fact is that my heart is not that great. I have this heart problem and everything else. I started to realize I only have, God knows, how many years—twenty at the most, if I live that long. If I kept going the way I was, I would not even make ten out of it. I would not even make retirement. I said I better do something about it. I had been thinking about doing something before. This time I made up my mind that I would do something about it.

The next morning, Dennis phoned the EHP for an appointment, and within a few days he was in a twenty-eight-day rehabilitation program.

When the supervisor's accommodation breaks down, the employee is forced into doing something to retain his or her job. There also appears, however, to be some interaction between supervisory discussions and cultural triggers. This was suggested in Dennis's case. He called attention to his drinking's interference with his health after first speaking of losing his job. The supervisor's remarks seem to set off the cultural triggering patterns. The cases of Elizabeth T. and Mary Margaret O. further illustrate this effect. Both women suffered from migraines for ten to fifteen years, and both had contained them with a wide variety of strategies and tactics. Both had considered biofeedback as a means of controlling their headaches, but neither had followed through until her supervisor discussed Corpco's biofeedback program with her. Both appeared to react to their supervisors' intervention within the confines of their respective cultural triggers. Mary Margaret O. seemed to express her rationale for coming in terms of sanctioning, and Elizabeth T. in terms of personal and family relations.

Mary Margaret:

Ok, the way it actually happened was when I started working for my new boss. I am sick with a migraine, and he suggested that I come to the health program and look into biofeedback. . . . A couple of people that I knew did say, "Did you ever think about going to biofeedback?" I would say, "Yes." But nobody really gave me a push, I guess, to really look into it.

Elizabeth:

My boss recommended it. Actually I had been thinking about it. . . . I really did not know if I qualified as being that desperately in need, so I just kept putting it off. But things got really bad in terms of headaches and things like that. When I would get it, it would be just horrible. So my boss one time said, "What is the matter?" We had been talking about it, and he said, "Why don't you try biofeedback?" . . . When my boss mentioned it, I thought to myself, "Hey, it has been a few years now. Maybe you are a real candidate for this thing. . . . And your husband is not too pleased to find you with a cold rag on your head. . . ." I think putting the cold rag on my head always turned me off anyway. . . . It just got to the point where, boy, if I can be helped, why am I sitting around living like this?

Company medical routines also induce employees to use the EHP. The many examinations conducted by the medical department are meant to keep employees in peak physical condition. Prevalent among these are the preemployment physical, the annual checkup, and such periodic examinations such as hypertension screening. All are offered on a routine basis. When hired, each employee undergoes a thorough medical examination. All employees are encouraged to have an annual physical; those over forty years of age are required to have one each year. Hypertension screening is available at all times, and, periodically, campaigns are waged to induce employees to take the tests. Employees who evidence abnormal blood pressure or heart problems are encouraged to use the screening service every three to four weeks to monitor their progress.

Such routines provide the medical program with a steady work flow and many opportunities to intervene in employees' lives. When examining physicians or nurses spot what they believe are troublesome conditions or behaviors, they make recommendations for altering them. Their recommendations vary from simple dietary advice and drug prescribing to referral for further professional consultation. One referral is to the EHP, and this typically occurs when the condition is perceived to have a behavioral component that has not been amenable to dietary or drug interventions. Medical routines also provide employees with the opportunity to air problems about which they are concerned but have not taken any action (e.g., Zola 1972). For example, Elizabeth T., who was encouraged to use biofeedback by her boss, did not know where to make the appointment. Consequently, she first phoned the medical department to set up her annual physical. During the examination, she asked the doctor about using biofeedback to control the migraines, and he referred her to the EHP. While providing information about biofeedback, this strategy also relieved Elizabeth of taking responsibility for the referral, since the doctor assured her she was an acceptable candidate for treatment. Her behavior was fairly typical of those employees who did not know that biofeedback was part of the EHP. But it obscures the employee's true motivation for referral, and the case is recorded in the EHP records as simply a medical referral, when in fact, it was often induced by one of the cultural triggers or a supervisory discussion.

Deborah F.'s case illustrates how preemployment physicals encourage referrals. Deborah had been working at Corpco for six months as a temporary employee. When a full-time secretarial position opened, she applied for and received it. Three years earlier, she was ill with the flu, and her doctor told her that she would have to quit smoking. She was unable to pay for smoking cessation classes at the Ford Foundation, the Cancer Society, or the Heart and Lung Association. She perceived that her smoking made her short-winded and that she had some difficulty climbing stairs.

Deborah:

> First, I had to have the usual company physical exam
> . . . so she was telling me then about also having the
> psychiatric section, the emotional health area, and she
> mentioned biofeedback. That is what alerted me to per-
> haps taking advantage of the service here as an employee.
> I made an appointment to see, to talk to, someone about
> biofeedback; plus my smoking concerns me.

In Deborah F.'s case, the perceived interference with physical functioning preceded the preemployment physical, which
provided her with the opportunity to do something about her
smoking. The interplay between medical routines and cultural triggers is further illustrated by Robert R.'s case. He
suffered a severe fall to which he attributed his elevated blood
pressure. He had always been physically active, playing football in high school, and he always expected to live as long as
his parents, who were now in their eighties. His sports activities had been curtailed due to his injured ankle and elevated
blood pressure. He was monitoring his blood pressure in Corpco's medical program and hoped to be playing sports again
soon:

> From that time, I have had a blood pressure problem. . . .
> I would have periods when it would elevate and then it
> would go back to normal, and I was getting readings
> consistently in the high normal range the last few weeks.
> I was always active physically. I like to play a lot of
> tennis. I used to jog some; I used to do a lot of swimming;
> and, then, after the accident I was limited in what I could
> do. . . . I wanted to take steps to bring it down into the
> normal range again. It was suggested that I try a salt-free
> diet, but I travel a lot, and that is very difficult at times.
> Also, there are a lot of pressures with the job, and you
> sit all day. It does not help if you do not get your proper
> exercise in. So I headed over to the blood pressure clinic,
> so it could be watched [and] so it would not get out of

> hand. Then, it started to rise even more, and . . . it was
> suggested would I want to consider biofeedback.

Robert was prompted to use the screening program because he perceived that his fractured ankle and elevated blood pressure interfered with his physical and vocational functioning. When testing revealed that diet alone could not contain his blood pressure and when he refused to take medication, Corpco's doctors referred him to the EHP for biofeedback.

Medical routines can induce employees to self-refer who would not otherwise do so. Lorraine P. had previously attributed her sleep problems to menopause, but conflict with her boss aggravated her tenseness and sleeplessness.

> This job problem came up the last week of April, the
> first week of May. I really was not sleeping. It was just
> at that time that I had the review. I do not think that I
> would have gone to the doctor for it. I probably would
> not have gone to Dr. Rose or my family doctor. But I
> was having the review, the annual checkup, and it came
> up at that point. I explained that I wake up and [that]
> my shoulders are so tense, they just ache. I could not
> get back to sleep. I was getting extremely tired. . . . If
> you do not sleep at night, you are going to be tired the
> next day. It just stands to reason. She said, "I think bio-
> feedback might be helpful and make an appointment
> with Jay and see if it is."

The workplace triggers appear to function differently for lower level employees and management-level employees. Among the program users I interviewed, employee networks and supervisory discussions induced lower level employees to refer themselves to the EHP; medical routines induced both lower and management-level employees to refer themselves to the EHP. The largest proportion of those encouraged to refer themselves by medical routines were managers.

Employee networks were involved in five referrals. All these cases involved lower level employees. It is not clear why employee networks are more likely to encourage lower level employees to refer themselves than to encourage management-level employees. Several factors may contribute to this tendency. First, managers appear to be better informed about the EHP's existence and how it works, a function of the EHP presentations that, until recently, were a regular part of the orientation and training of new managers. Second, management-level employees may be more reluctant to consult others about their problems than lower-level employees are, and third, managers who did consult the employee network before referral may have self-selected themselves out of the interviews.

Supervisory discussions were involved in six cases, and all these cases involved lower level employees. This finding parallels Harrison Trice and Janice Beyer's findings that supervisory referrals for alcoholism in a government employee assistance program are predominantly lower level employees (1977). Again, there are several possible explanations for this phenomenon. First, lower level employees are probably more susceptible to supervisory discussions than management-level employees because they are more closely supervised. While lower level employees usually perform routine tasks in open areas under the watchful gaze of their supervisors, the manager typically performs his or her tasks within an office protected by a secretary. Consequently, lower level employees are more visible and more susceptible to interventions than managers are. Second, when managers are confronted either formally or informally by their supervisors, they may possess greater resources than lower level employees have for resisting an EHP referral. For example, they may follow through with a referral to an outside helping agent or agency, whereas lower level employees cannot afford that option.

Medical routines were involved in eight cases. Of these, three involved lower level employees and five involved management-level employees. In this instance, the proportion of management employees probably reflects the greater utilization of routine medical services by higher level employees.

Most managers have an annual examination because most of these upper level employees are over the age of forty and therefore required to do so. I suspect that one reason medical routines induce managers to refer themselves is that managers find it difficult to counter medical expertise. This is to suggest not that managers do not seek ways of avoiding compliance with the advice but that managers find it more difficult to evade medical opinion than to evade either coworker or supervisory recommendations. Managers usually checked the Corpco physician's recommendation for biofeedback treatment with their family doctor or family members, who typically stated that it could not hurt and usually encouraged them to give it a try. Such support combined with the manager's lack of medical expertise makes it difficult for him or her not to comply.

Point of entry

The discussion of triggers and workplace structures reveals that employees enter the EHP via two avenues. They refer themselves either directly to the EHP or indirectly through the medical department. Thirteen employees referred themselves directly to the EHP, and seventeen referred themselves indirectly through the medical department. Table 4.1 shows the point of entry by cultural triggers and workplace struc-

TABLE 4.1
Point of Entry to the Emotional Health Program,
by Cultural Triggers and Workplace Structures

	Through Medical Program	Directly to EHP	Total
Cultural triggers	7	3	10
Medical routines	8	0	8
Supervisory discussions	2	4	6
Employee networks	0	6	6
Total	17	13	30

tures. What accounts for these differences? Knowledge of the EHP's existence and services appears to explain the difference in entry points. Those employees who were knowledgeable about the program and its services usually referred themselves directly to the EHP, and those who had no such knowledge referred themselves via the medical program. Employee networks and supervisory discussions were instrumental in supplying employees with such knowledge, and they were involved in ten of the thirteen direct referrals to the EHP. In seven of these cases of direct referral, this contact was the first time that the employee had ever heard of the EHP and its services. In the remaining six cases of direct referral, the employee knew of the EHP through Corpco literature or the grapevine or previous use. Generally those employees who were referred through the medical program did not know of the EHP's existence and its services. This was also true of those employees who referred themselves to the medical program because of supervisory discussions. In the supervisory cases, neither the employee nor the supervisor knew that the alcoholism and biofeedback programs were located within the EHP.

A second distinction can be made between employees who were referred to the medical department and those directly referred to the EHP. Generally those employees who referred themselves to the medical department did so because they perceived that their problems were physical and required the services of a physician; those employees who referred themselves to the EHP, whether they perceived their problems as physical or emotional or both, saw themselves as requiring psychological services. This points up the great importance of employee networks and supervisory discussions in helping employees to define their problems. Through such interactions the employee recognizes that his or her problem can be alleviated by behavioral interventions and learns to present his or her problem to the EHP in that manner. By contrast, employees who refer themselves to the medical program learn these things from their interaction with Corpco's physicians and nurses. Consequently, these workplace structures perform an important function in educating employees about the EHP and its use, a function analogous to what Charles Kadushin (1969) has termed the "friends and supporters of psychotherapy." However, Kadushin's "friends" are former users of private psychotherapy in the general community, whereas these structures are specific to the workplace and the EHP.

Final decisions

Before the employee actually refers himself or herself to the EHP, several final decisions must be made. These final decisions involve the factors found to influence utilization of medical facilities (chapter 2): What is the expense? How convenient is the service? Does the EHP use drugs? Is the service confidential?

Expense is a concern to employees only when they consider the use of alternative services. Indeed, all take for granted that Corpco's medical services are free to employees, and all tend to rely upon the medical department to provide their routine care (e.g., colds), because it is less costly than using an outside practitioner, and on their family doctor or a specialist primarily for nonroutine health care (e.g., a broken arm). Both those employees who report having a family doctor and those who report not having one use Corpco's services. Many of the employees report warm feelings for Corpco's physicians. Comments such as, "I wish Dr. Rose could be my regular family doctor" were fairly typical. Consequently, the decision to refer oneself to the medical program is both familiar and easy, especially when the services are free.

Expense is of more concern for employees considering the EHP than for those considering the medical department, because usually neither the counseling staff nor the behavioral interventions are personally known to the employees. Consequently, many do consider alternative psychological services. But very quickly they begin to realize that they have even less information about alternatives, since few if any of their acquaintances or family have ever used such services, and that even with their insurance coverage, outside services remain fairly expensive. Expense is especially troublesome to employees when they still have to be convinced of the therapy's efficacy. The opportunity to experiment with unfamiliar techniques without financial cost is particularly attractive. As Diana D. states,

> This is a good place to start, because by coming here I could find out if something like this might help, without the financial burden. If you went outside and you paid someone, you might find that this really was not helping that much and all that money would have gone down the drain.

For many employees, like Norman B., the fact that the EHP's services are free means the difference between obtaining and not obtaining professional advice.

> The only [other] place I would have gone was my doctor. But other than that? Ok, be honest! Go to a doctor and sit in his office for an hour and talk. Sure! My paycheck would be going to him and the rest would be going upstate. I would be eating bread and water on the corner. No, if this was not here, I would still be trying to talk it out with myself, my folks, and the girl.

Convenience is also of concern to employees. They appreciate being able to receive help during working hours. Frequently, the alternative is taking a half day off from work, and, for hourly workers, this means lost income. Using the company program means they do not have to worry about such scheduling difficulties. As one employee states, "It is so easy. I come down here, and I am back in an hour." It is also easy because employees must tell their supervisor only that they have an appointment with the medical department, whereas if they have an appointment with an outside practitioner, they frequently must provide more elaborate excuses for being absent.

103

While expense and convenience were important consider-
ations for employees, these concerns were much less important than those of drug use and confidentiality. Again and
again in the interviews, employees stated that their decision
to refer themselves was based on assurances that the program
would teach them to control their problems without the use
of drugs. For many, this concern stemmed from previous unpleasant experiences in which a drug made them "feel like a
zombie"; in general, these individuals recounted medical his-
tories of noncompliance. Others considered drug taking to be
a drastic solution for what they believed were problems still
solvable by less dramatic methods. Closely allied to this idea
were beliefs that drug use inevitably leads to dependency and
indicates the problem is beyond individual control. Repeat-
edly, employees stated that they "were not that sick," that
they "did not want to become dependent upon drugs," and
that they wanted to control their own behavior. Assurances
from the medical staff, coworkers, and supervisors that the
EHP did not rely upon drugs were an important factor in
employees' decisions to refer themselves.

Confidentiality is the issue of greatest concern to employees. They fear the reactions of others should their involvement with the EHP become known, and specifically they fear
that, if management should discover their involvement, their
careers would be jeopardized. Confidentiality is an issue for
all of Corpco's medical programs. One Corpco vice president
estimates that "nearly two out of every three employees el-
igible for physical examinations do not use them because they
fear management will see their files." This suggests that those
who use the medical department do have confidence in the
department's ability to maintain confidentiality. When asked
about the EHP's ability to maintain confidentiality, one employee responded, "I assumed it was confidential because it
was part of the medical department." Previous personal experiences with the medical department, as well as the assurances of employee network members, supervisors, and referring
physicians, appear to be important factors in convincing em-

104

ployees of the EHP's ability to maintain confidentiality. Despite these repeated assurances, often the first questions asked by employees when they arrive for the EHP intake interview concern confidentiality. Diana D.'s comment is typical.

> The only real question I had was that I wanted to be confident that all my records would be confidential, because I did not want it on my employee record. . . . I got it straightened out right away in my mind that, in fact, the records were confidential.

In the end, confidentiality determines whether the employee ultimately goes to the EHP and confides in the therapist. Free and accessible services encourage the employee to refer himself or herself. But the manner in which confidentiality is handled by the medical and emotional health programs can easily discourage the employee from referring himself or herself, and confidentiality remains an issue even after he or she leaves the program.

What the referral decision means

Troubled employees become aware of themselves as possessing undesirable attributes, and they believe that, should these attributes become known to their coworkers, supervisors, and management, they will become discredited. Consequently, they engage in a variety of strategies and tactics to contain information about these discreditable attributes. Through selective conversations with others, they learn that their problems are normal and containable. The containment phase is broken by symptoms, cultural triggers, which are learned rationales for referral, and workplace triggers that constitute the reactions of others.

The cultural triggers appear to be transmitted from generation to generation by family and kinship networks, and they probably constitute part of "what everybody knows." These triggers permit the individual to reflect upon his or her own situation and decide whether to refer to a professional practitioner. In this instance, the individual is reacting to his or her socialization and exercising self-control. But self-control over what? Essentially, the individual is not trying to gain control over physical or emotional distress but to regain control over difficult social relationships. In a sense, the individual presents biological problems in order to relieve social difficulties. As Talcott Parsons (1951) suggested many years ago, there is a secondary gain for individuals who assume the sick role and put themselves in the hands of a physician. This is particularly true of those individuals who refer themselves to the program because of an interpersonal crisis—they seek a medical escape from their social ordeals. Those who refer themselves because they perceive that their symptoms either interfere or are about to interfere with their personal relationships, work, or physical functioning seek medical advice in order to prevent further deterioration and to regain control over these spheres of their lives. Those who refer themselves because of sanctions seek medical advice in order to comply with the reactions of others who have taken the responsibility of deciding that containment has broken down.

The referral process revealed by employee interviews is a distinctly social process, a process in which employees are aware of their own discreditable attributes and react to those attributes on the basis of previously acquired knowledge and the reactions of family, coworkers, supervisors, and medical personnel. Through these interactions employees build a concept of their problems as amenable to medical interventions and decide to refer themselves. Indeed, the decision to refer oneself to the EHP results from a complex interaction of both formal and informal social controls. Throughout this process, however, it is not the individual's discreditable attribute that changes and leads to the referral decision. Rather, a change in the individual as she or he reflects upon the attribute or a change in the significant audience leads to the referral decision.

5. Diagnosis and therapy

This chapter explores the manner in which the staff react to and treat employees who use the emotional health program. I pay special attention to how organizational factors and the staff's occupational roles affect the creation of diagnoses and the treatment of employees, and by exploring this process, I am focusing on some of the ways in which the EHP orders and mediates the relationship between the individual employee and Corpco. In this context, the EHP staff are the company's agents of control, who perform the "dirty work" (Hughes 1962) of containing and regulating the offending elements of employees' behavior while shielding other workers from contamination by those elements.

I use the term therapist to mean the interns and the consulting psychologists who collectively provide psychotherapy to employees; however, when it is necessary to identify the specific group, I use the terms interns and consulting psychologists. Likewise, I use the term EHP director to mean both the former director (the clinical psychologist) and the current director (the psychiatrist), but I also speak of each separately. Since the therapists think of the case records as their personal notes, they write their comments in abbreviated form: they write incomplete sentences, drop articles, insert shorthand symbols, and jump from thought to thought. In reconstructing the case records, I have completed sentences, inserted articles, translated symbols, and attempted to clarify thoughts. I have made every effort to retain the therapist's intent; however, I have edited out information that I believe would jeopardize an employee's anonymity.

In setting goals for its EHP, Corpco provides the context in which the EHP treats employees. Because Corpco and its EHP are in transition, however, goals are not always clear. But when questioned, the staff state that the program is generally expected to provide short-term therapy for employees, save the company money, and keep the work force productive. The following response from a therapist is typical:

> I would assume that it was to increase productivity on the part of the employee. . . . The people that we were seeing were having difficulty in functioning in their performance, sometimes only on the job, sometimes both at home and on the job. And we were trying in some way to alleviate the reasons, the problems, that were causing the difficulties they were having.

According to the director, management expects the EHP to operate on a number of levels, and it is the program director's job to interpret at which level the management expects it to be operating at any given moment.

> I do not get a clear message which level they [management] are operating on, when. Ideally, from upper management's point of view, there is an idealistic, humanistic venture involved, as well as productivity. From a middle management point of view, there is a productivity issue involved, and from a medical-legal point of view there is a protect-the-company issue involved. So all those things are kind of operating simultaneously. . . . I have to respond to all those levels at all times. . . . depending on what mood everybody in the business is in, because there is tremendous filtration down. You know, if [the chairman] is going to Washington, the humanitarian interests go way up. If [the vice president of human resources management] is going to visit, the productivity and nonsense issues go way up.

In the final analysis, the program's direction is based on top management's demands and not upon the staff's psychiatric ideology and expertise. This point was dramatically driven home when Corpco's chairman ordered the EHP director to resurrect the company's alcoholism program because he felt employees were drinking too much. The current director described this reality.

> In terms of getting real support, the president of the corporation has to like it. Because he liked alcoholism, he spent, God knows, the cost of the alcoholism task force, to redo what we already had. . . . We rewrote the manual and procedural outline. . . . They're much more up-to-date with an out-of-date idea. You know, alcoholism as a separate entity. . . . We're trying to get our foot in the troubled-employee door. . . . But that is not the direction [in which he wants to go]. He wanted an alcoholism thing. That [idea] was 10 years ago.

The former director added that, as a result of the refocus on alcoholism, "We are going to be working on increasing management referrals. . . . That is one of [the chairman's] mandates for 1982."

The most contentious issue surrounding the EHP is whether its purpose should be to deliver short-term psychotherapy or referral services. That is, should Corpco's therapists be providing employees with treatment in ten fifty-minute sessions or simply be referring them to psychotherapists outside of the company after a maximum of three sessions. A therapist explained that this controversy evolved from a report written by the former director:

> Initially, it [short-term therapy] was considered cost-effective because [the director] had done a study to that effect. And he had worked out a formula for how he converted workers' time and the effect of a disturbed or troubled person on all the other employees, and he worked that out in dollars and cents. And he came out with this

plan that, if you treated people right on the job, that then this ripple effect was cut off, and therefore everyone worked better. More harmoniously. And productivity was greater. And the company saved money. And there was an actual formula for that. And the debate then came to rest on the fact that the company also provided such a generous insurance policy for its own employees that high-quality care was available outside the company. And the ripple effect kind of was disregarded. There were people who did not believe [his] formula. Like his boss. . . . His boss was very adamant about the fact that he [the boss] thought it should be an even shorter term service, that people should only be seen three times, and that beyond that it was an overlap, that it was no longer cost-efficient.

Concerns that Corpco could be sued for malpractice if an employee was unsatisfied with his or her treatment add legal fuel to this treatment-referral controversy. The current director stated,

If I were advising the president, I would have them not do any primary care because of the economic dangers to the company in terms of lawsuits. Which is the ugly state I find medicine in. That it is not in their interest to take any responsibility whatsoever for anybody. . . . Refer them out, sure. Let somebody else get sued, until something changes and you can afford a $2-million lawsuit.

Although generally the EHP director protects the interns from management's conflicting demands and arbitrariness and encourages them to see their role as clinical, the treatment-referral controversy disturbs them deeply because it directly threatens their clinical role. Indeed, the interns question whether doing simple referral will satisfy their internship requirements and see it in their self-interest to do short-term therapy. Consequently, they characterize management as not understanding and desiring "miracle therapy." As one therapist commented about the manager who rejected the cost-effectiveness of short-term therapy,

> From my point of view, he had very little concept of process in emotional health. So he seemed to think that a person could sit down and tell you their problem, and magically there would be a resolution, and the person would feel great. And that it was the contact that did it. He did not seem to understand therapy as a process. So, in effect, what he was advocating could only be a referral service.

The therapists rejected the notion of a referral service and Corpco's definition of short-term therapy as well, preferring to define short-term as eight months to a year.

> I think [private practice] offers a chance to pursue different modalities without the restrictions that the company puts on. Like we were told at Corpco in the beginning, we should not see people more than ten times. But maybe twenty was OK. And now it is three. Well, people do not always have problems that work out on Corpco's timetable.

Consequently, the therapists carried employees for as long as possible. Indeed, two reported working with employees for a year, and a third says, "Most of the clients that I saw took more than ten sessions."

Multiple mandates and autonomy

Social control agents often feel conflict about their roles because of the multiplicity of goals they are expected to pursue or implement (Schur 1979). Such feelings can be particularly difficult for professionals, who prize autonomy as a symbol of their status (Freidson 1970). Other researchers (Daniels 1969 and 1972, Halleck 1972, Szasz 1970) have illustrated the extent to which the psychiatric role is confounded by a mixture of therapeutic and control functions, which create ambiguous feelings in therapists. To overcome such feelings usually means that the therapists must adapt to the organization's goals. Arlene Daniels, discussing military psychiatrists, noted that

> for a successful bureaucratic adaptation, professionals need to develop a primary commitment to the larger aims or general rationale of the organizations they serve. . . . And he may not feel that he is a captive of the organization as he goes about his work. (1969, 264)

The EHP staff initially expressed concern about pursuing the dual mandates of therapy and control and perceived them as a conflict of interest that threatened their professional autonomy: on the one hand, they saw the pursuit of therapy as supporting the employee and as being the ethical professional choice; on the other hand, they saw the pursuit of control as supporting the organization against the employee and as being unethical and unprofessional. Unlike their military counterparts, who resolve the issue by perceiving the organization as their client (Daniels 1969 and 1972), the therapists maintain that the employee is their client. One therapist commented,

> I was very skeptical when I first came here. How can you possibly do a patient any good when you are supposed to be working for the company, which could be doing strange things to the patient? That conflict-of-interest sort of thing.

To the therapist's great relief, "that has not been a problem at all." As one therapist explained, the conflict is resolved in the employee's favor because the company allows the therapists to perform their work autonomously.

> I was empowered to do my job fully and given the autonomy to make decisions as if I were in private practice. So that I was resolved—absolved, almost—from the ethical conflict of what do we do if the company would

benefit from one thing and the client would benefit from another. It resolved in favor always of the client.

Indeed, all the therapists perceive that when they "close the door" to their consulting rooms, they are "relatively free" to focus upon the employee's needs and to recommend the most appropriate therapy. Several factors support their perception of autonomy: selectivity, alternative statuses, lack of close supervision, and enforcement of confidentiality.

Unlike their military counterparts, who are drafted into the service (Daniels 1969 and 1972), Corpco's therapists are se-lected into the company based upon special criteria. To the extent that Corpco is able to select therapists whose interests coincide with those of the company, it is able to allow them to exercise a greater degree of control over their work. At any given time, there are more interns and consulting psycholo-gists seeking to work for Corpco than there are therapy po-sitions; the EHP received several hundred resumés for the part-time opening that was filled during my research, and the program director received telephone inquiries about employ-ment opportunities throughout this period. Consequently, the company is able to match very closely its interests to those of its therapists. Interns who are accepted into the program are generally older students (thirty to thirty-five years old) with some clinical experience. Corpco considers such stu-dents mature enough to understand "the special needs" of work organizations (i.e., not disrupt the company's work). And, finally, as the former director states, all therapists ac-cepted into the program are interested in learning about, and working within, the EHP's short-term treatment framework:

> If the program emphasis is short-term, cognitive-be-havioral orientation, what this means is that any intern coming into our program is going to be taught in that unique modality. It also means that any staff member will be expected to follow up with that treatment ap-proach. So, with respect to the types of treatment and types of practitioners, there are going to be those lim-

> itations. . . . If a therapist here would like to do long-term treatment, this really is not the place for them. . . . If a person cannot in some way integrate themselves into the corporate culture, of which they are a part, then, here again, this is not the place for them. I would say that the constraints are few, but meaningful in terms of their implications. If you do not feel like wearing a suit and tie every day, this really is not the place for you.

Despite concerns about the number of sessions, the interns and the consulting psychologists appear fairly content within the EHP's limitations. Indeed, the interns consider their Corpco internship "a plum" that is providing them with a valuable clinical experience and entry to future industrial employment opportunities. One therapist says candidly,

> From my vantage point, looking at the market situation for psychologists, I did not see any situation that would provide better working conditions and a better salary. I think it is an exciting kind of practice. Many of my colleagues are working in mental health agencies [where they] suffer real occupational hazards. Callousness. Burnout. . . . And it [Corpco] offers a tremendous opportunity to get more of a national scope. Flying here and there for meetings and conventions. Most people do not have access to that. To me it is appealing. I like this kind of life.

Judging from these remarks, the rewards for those therapists who can adapt to the corporate culture and work within the short-term modality are high. The rewards for the consulting psychologists are different but equally rewarding. Their consulting work provides them opportunities to be with colleagues and with opportunities to expand their expertise by learning first-hand about "the problems of people in the workplace."

Because Corpco is able to exercise selectivity in hiring, choosing clinicians whose interests coincide with its program's objectives, it permits those clinicians to pursue their work with a high degree of autonomy. This freedom is corroborated by the fact that therapists work at Corpco part time and therefore must have alternative forms of support. Having an alternative status (e.g., student, private practitioner) seems to increase the degree of autonomy that therapists experience. This is particularly true of the consulting psychologists, who have successful private practices and are not completely dependent upon Corpco for their livelihoods. Indeed one psychologist spoke of his "fees doubling in private practice" and having "the luxury of not being a staff person and therefore remaining outside of the conflicts." Unlike psychologists, interns are not paid, but being unpaid affords its own sense of freedom. As one intern remarked, "That [being unpaid and a student] gave us a freedom that we would not have had on the payroll." In effect, being off the payroll, they felt free to focus on the individual employee as their client.

The interns' sense of autonomy is also enhanced by the fact that they were not closely supervised by either the former or current EHP director. This is a result of the directors' philosophies (i.e., give people freedom and they will perform) and of the time constraints placed upon the directors' own work. The current director is at Corpco only two or three days a week. The former director, who is busy with his new job, no longer has day-to-day contact with the interns, but remains involved because their internships require that they be supervised by a state-certified psychologist. Consequently, the interns are free from close supervision, and, to a great degree, they interact with the current and former director only when they need technical advice on a particular case and at the regularly scheduled training sessions and case reviews. They are relatively free to focus on individual employees who seek their advice and to determine their own diagnoses and treatment plans.

Confidentiality

Confidentiality regulations shield therapists' work from the view of others. Regulations govern access to the employee's emotional health case record and the information that therapists may share with those who inquire about the employee's involvement in the EHP. Therapists consider emotional health records to be their personal notes, and they restrict access to them. One therapist remarked that,

> as far as I am concerned, the psychiatric record that we keep on the patient is strictly between the patient and me. And nobody else. . . . unless the patient writes the consent and says that it is acceptable.

Until recently, the case records were kept in the medical file where the employee, physician, and nurse practitioners had access to them. In November 1980, the Occupational Health and Safety Administration (OSHA) ruled that an employee's representative (e.g., union steward) was also to have access to the medical files, and at the same time, OSHA mandated that, if drug abuse and mental health records were kept separate from medical records, they were not accessible to union stewards. Although Corpco was not unionized, the program director used this ruling as an excuse to create a separate psychiatric file that restricts access to everyone, including Corpco's physicians and nurse practitioners, without the employee's written consent. In addition, under the new procedure, the employee is not permitted to review his or her psychiatric file without his or her therapist present. The EHP claimed this precaution is necessary because employees are apt to misinterpret the notes without the therapist's help. While this procedure assures the employee's privacy, it also increases the control therapists have over their work by ensuring that no one has access to the only written record describing the therapist's diagnosis and treatment plan. My own experience reviewing these case records attests that the EHP vigilantly restricts access to them. All requests without both the employee's written consent and the director's approval are routinely denied.

The therapists share as little information as possible with anyone asking about an employee's involvement with the EHP. As a matter of course, the program rejects all such requests without the employee's written consent. Most often such inquiries are from an employee's supervisor, who wishes to know if the person has been to the EHP as reported. The program perceives such inquiries as jeopardizing an employee's privacy and drawing the therapists toward the control side of their multiple mandate. The program uses several strategies to preserve its clinical focus. First, it informs such supervisors that they may call the medical desk to confirm whether an employee has been to the medical department, but that they will receive no information about what programs he or she is using. If a supervisor seeks information beyond that, the therapists respond that all such information is confidential. All the therapists reported having had to confront such supervisors at one time or another. The following comment from a therapist was typical:

> I would have to say [to the supervisor], "I'm really not at liberty to discuss that with you." And I think most supervisors understood that and appreciated it. There were some who were really looking for a weapon, and they would try and push and push. But we were clearly told, "You do not give any information."

On occasion, a supervisor does manage to bulldoze his or her way beyond this line of defense. When this happens, the therapist counters with a splitting strategy in which a second therapist meets with the supervisor and discusses in general how to manage a "troubled" employee. One therapist reported such an episode:

> One supervisor in particular was brought in to me. . . . I was seeing a patient, and, one day, one of the medical doctors brought over this patient's supervisor to meet

117

with me and talk about the patient. . . . And I said, "Hold it! I can't do that." And the only way they could appease the supervisor was to have her meet with another counselor, who would then discuss with her how you handle an employee generally who demonstrates these qualities. . . . And that was really a result, I think, of the medical people. It was something that we would never have done.

My interviews and observations suggest to me that the staff have been very successful in resisting all demands to share information and that this success has increased their sense of autonomy and has preserved their focus upon the individual employee. The question remains, however, whether or not they are really able to resolve all conflicts of interest in the employee's favor. Indeed, such psychiatric mavericks as Thomas Szasz (1961) and R. D. Laing (1965) contend that social control is intrinsic to psychiatric practice and that diagnoses and treatment almost always incorporate elements of control. Therapists must often implicitly "take sides" in situations of interpersonal conflict, even if they "habitually conceal and mystify their partisanship behind a cloak of therapeutic neutrality, never admitting to being either the patient's ally or his adversary" (Szasz 1970, 71; see also Halleck 1972; Schur 1979).

A social-control function is intrinsic to the short-term cognitive-behavioral therapies used in Corpco's EHP. In fact, these therapies require that the therapist focus upon the individual employee and emphasize the employee's responsibility for doing something about his or her own problem. This automatically absolves the organization of any responsibility for an employee's problem and shifts the burden to the individual. For example, when employees complain of work stress, such therapy emphasizes their "abnormal" reactions to "normal" stress and teaches them to respond more "appropriately." Although such a procedure cannot ignore completely the organizational demands, it does help to minimize an employee's concern with them. By focusing upon the employee and away from the organization, therapists exercise control in the company's behalf. Hiring therapists who are comfortable with this approach means that such control can be exercised while assuring the therapists of a high level of autonomy. As one therapist said, "This is my brand of psychotherapy. My approach. So, as long as I am consistent with that, I do not feel that there are any conflicts."

One way to reveal the social control functions intrinsic to Corpco's therapies is to investigate how much discretion the therapists have in working with employees. In this examination, discretion is defined as "the freedom or authority to make decisions and to choose from among possible processing actions" (Schur 1979, 350).

Creating a diagnosis

Diagnosis is a major element in every therapist's work, and each employee who uses the EHP has a diagnosis listed on his or her emotional health record. This diagnosis was previously based upon those listed in the ninth edition of the *International Classification of Diseases* (*ICD*-9), but it is currently based upon the third edition of the *Diagnostic and Statistical Manual* (*DSM*-III). The EHP switched diagnostic manuals because *DSM*-III is more behaviorally oriented than the psychoanalytically oriented *ICD*-9. The practical implications of this are that patients, instead of being diagnosed as having an anxiety neurosis or obsessive neurosis are diagnosed as having an anxiety reaction or compulsive disorder, labels that are thought to be more descriptive and less stigmatizing than the old diagnoses.

Theoretically, the purpose of a diagnosis is to describe accurately an individual's problem so that it can be matched with an appropriate form of treatment. The construction of a diagnosis is based on the process of retrospective interpretation (Schur 1971), whereby the therapist "rereads" the char-

119

acter of the employee. This process, described here by a Corpco therapist, entails the use of progressively fewer and fewer details about the employee until the therapist has uncovered the "essential problem":

> You elicit responses to initially a wide variety of basic questions in the classic intake interview, and then you begin to narrow down through questioning. Once you have heard, let us say, that they are finding it difficult to sleep and they are having crying spells and they are beginning to feel hopeless, then you begin to focus in on depression. Or if, for example, they are having free-floating fears, you try to get more specific with that. But it starts with the basic intake interview and then goes to a more specific level of eliciting the symptoms and finally to the arena of the specific diagnosis.

Although many researchers (e.g., Goffman 1961; Rosenhan 1973; Scheff 1968; and Schur 1971 and 1979) question the meaning and accuracy of psychiatric diagnoses, the program director believes that "they are more accurate now that they are based on *DSM*-III types of protocols." Despite such disclaimers, uncertainty in creating diagnoses is a general feature of medicine (Conrad 1976; Mechanic 1968), and it remains a problem for the EHP therapists. Renee Fox (1957) delineates two types of uncertainty: uncertainty from personal inadequacy (or lack of training) and uncertainty from the limits of medical knowledge. Both types are present in the EHP. For example, several Corpco physicians initially questioned whether interns were sufficiently trained to diagnose and treat employees, and the interns themselves voiced such concerns:

> I was hesitant about doing that at first because I felt, number one, my background was not that good where I was really sure of a diagnosis without consulting someone. So I was a little hesitant to write on someone's record, you know, "manic depressive."

Likewise, the therapists express the beliefs that diagnosis is limited by current knowledge and that in the future diagnoses will be more accurate:

> I think, given the present state of the art (I do not think psychology is a science). . . . we are beginning to make major breakthroughs. . . . All kinds of interesting stuff that really clearly differentiate people who are suffering from certain psychiatric disorders from the mainstream. . . . I certainly hope that the next generation of psychologists and psychiatrists will have far more accurate indices. I am certain that they will look at our stuff the way we look on the old timers that preceded us. They seem very primitive.

Corpco's therapists employ several strategies to minimize uncertainty in diagnosis: multiple diagnoses, medical screening, and case reviews. The interns often record several diagnoses on the employee's case record, with the hope that future meetings with the employee will reduce their dilemma. One intern explained this procedure:

> I often start out, when I am not sure, really quite vague, I set down like three or four things, you know, written down in the psychiatric record after my entry. And then, when I see the person a second time, review those, keep in mind different facts, different things, that I saw that might do. But with some patients you do have two or three components. . . . In fact, it is rarely just one thing.

The therapists use medical examinations in order to assure themselves that the employee is suffering from a psychological problem and not a physiological one.

> The interface between physical problems and emotional problems is very hard to tease out, and diagnosis is essential in those areas. We need to know if someone has a brain tumor, and that is why they are hearing voices

—or if they are hallucinating because they are schizophrenic, and it is more of an emotional process. And that is where a diagnosis, to me, is really essential. . . . My training as a therapist, and my own perception of how I work, is that I would require a full exam before I would take on a patient.

Once a week the EHP director reviews with each intern the cases that he or she is handling. According to the former director, this reduces the interns' uncertainty by assuring them of the appropriateness of their diagnoses:

I think that you are still going to have some interrater differences [in diagnoses] based on experience, based on training, based on what sorts of issues come up in that specific interview. This is one of the reasons why we, of course, supervise our people closely, and we also want to assure that the diagnostician is . . . also the treating party. So that there is that consistency.

Despite the efforts to reduce uncertainty, a great deal of ambiguity about the meaning of the diagnosis remains. For example, the EHP director was skeptical about multiple diagnoses written on the case records: "When you see three diagnoses, forget it. Three diagnoses is no diagnosis." He recommended that interns use the terminology "diagnosis deferred," and one therapist remarked,

I do not think you can find a pure diagnostic statement. I think we see a mixed bag of symptomology. You can always make the case that you have a primary diagnosis with secondary features. That kind of shelters us from appearing like asses because we do not have the expertise.

In the end, all of the therapists agree that "one word does not describe a person very well."

One measure of the therapists' discomfort with diagnostic labels is their reluctance to share them with employees:

There is no value in it. You can communicate the same relevant information without a label that might be misconstrued or misused. When somebody attaches a label it takes on a shape of its own. Described problems or issues can be worked with, but a label is something that you can not do something about.

One therapist remarked, "I had a patient who was definitely paranoid. I think if I had told him he was paranoid, he would have killed me." Another asserted that "none of those candid sorts of conversations take place until there is some kind of relationship between the two of us and until I am confident that they can use it appropriately." The shift to diagnosis according to the *DSM*-III might make the therapists less reluctant to share such information with employees, but given the therapists' high level of reluctance to share information, I doubt that diagnoses will be shared more freely.

Why, then, does the EHP require the diagnosis? My interviews implied that diagnoses were created largely to demonstrate that something professional was being done about the employee's problem (Trice and Beyer 1981b) and to justify the therapists' actions (Goffman 1961). As one therapist speculated,

> The only reason I could see to diagnose was either for legal protection, if somebody got sued and you had to say what your diagnosis was, or for research. But I did not feel that, if either of those questions were ever called, that we really were sufficiently trained in fine-tooth diagnosis.

Another therapist pointed out that anxiety is often present in individuals who come to the program and that in order "to justify a medical intervention" in the case of a distraught woman whose husband had left her, he "would label [her] an adjustment reaction to depression." These comments suggest that diagnosis is largely a symbolic act to legitimate treatment. This justification is required by the employee, Corpco

123

management, and the interns' schools, and the case records function to prove that the therapists are acting professionally.

Processing stereotypes

If diagnosis is largely a symbolic act to justify medical interventions, how then do therapists make treatment decisions? The social constructionist literature suggests that control agents use processing stereotypes to make such decisions (Hawkins and Tiedeman 1975). The term processing stereotype encompasses the analytic concepts of "normal crimes" (Sudnow 1965) and "diagnostic stereotypes" (Scheff 1966), and it stresses the importance of standardized responses for diagnosis, prognosis, and treatment of individuals passing through social control agencies. Processing stereotypes, then, are simplified images used by social control agents to categorize and order their work.

The EHP uses four processing stereotypes in order to manage its work: true emergencies, false emergencies, standard routines, and variable routines (see table 5.1). These stereotypes emerge from the program's requirement to treat em-

TABLE 5.1
Processing Stereotypes, by Type of Referral and Treatment Choice

Treatment Choice	Emergency Referral	Routine Referral
Short-term therapy in the EHP	*False emergency*	*Standard routine*
Referral to outside treatment resource	*True emergency*	*Variable routine*

Note: The processing stereotypes were created in the following manner. First, in speaking of emergency referrals, the EHP staff differentiated between true emergencies and false emergencies. Therefore, true emergencies and false emergencies are a straight rendition of the staff's terminology. However, in speaking of employees who are not emergency referrals, the staff simply speak of "referrals," "clients," or "patients." Consequently the terminology "standard routines" and "variable routines" emerged from my observations of, and interviews with, the staff.

ployees within ten sessions and the notion of what constitutes a good candidate for short-term therapy. One therapist succinctly states the operating rule in processing employees through the program:

> It was really just a preliminary diagnosis . . . mainly to decide [whether] we felt this patient could be treated in the short-term situation or [whether] they should be referred out.

Unlike long-term therapy, which is generally psychoanalytically oriented and assumes that patients have an underlying character disorder, short-term therapy is behaviorally oriented and directed at immediate symptom relief. According to a Corpco therapist,

> Short-term therapy is centered on concrete problems. And that is one of the differences between being in psychoanalysis and being in short-term therapy, where you want relief of the symptoms. And so a person may present with five problems. And they tell you that number one and two are the most important. So you work on number one and number two, and when those are taken care of, you do not go into numbers three, four, and five. In long-term analysis you would. You work in terms of the whole person.

The former director further clarified this distinction:

> I would refer to so many of the psychiatric and psychological symptoms as just that. As symptoms and as problems in living. . . . With problems in living, people come in, and you teach them some skills and work with them to learn how to cope better in living in the world, and then they come back two, three, four years later at a time when they might once again be overwhelmed with their problems. . . . We have to appreciate that many illnesses, as well as the psychological problems in living, go through a natural course. . . . For example, I would

125

> suggest that the dimension of starting out with mild anxiety and ending up with what might be diagnosed as schizophrenia is a single dimension. . . . Depending upon where you fall on any one of these dimensions, I would make the distinction of illness versus a psychological symptom and a problem in living.

Short-term therapy, then, is perceived of as doing something about an employee's problem before it becomes an illness and requires some form of long-term therapy (e.g., psychoanalysis, hospitalization, surgery). The ideal candidate for short-term therapy is someone who comes to the EHP seeking help for a specific problem (e.g., migraine headaches, interpersonal relationships) and is highly motivated to do something about it.

Motivation is a key criterion in identifying the good candidate because, ideally, the program treats people in ten sessions or less. Therapists impute motivation to employees based upon the manner in which they enter the program. Employees who enter the program as emergency referrals are considered to be poorly motivated and are characterized as being out of control. Employees who enter the program as routine referrals are considered to be highly motivated and characterized as being in control of their behavior.

The term emergency connotes that something is out of control. This connotation was conveyed in one distraught employee's response to the medical receptionist who answered her phone call:

> When they said, "Is it an emergency?" I said that I was not going berserk, "I'm just asking for an appointment for your next available time. . . ." You do not want to say it is immediate and crucial. . . . You do not want people to think that you are cracking. . . . Obviously, if you are calling, it is crucial.

Indeed, as one therapist explained, the medical receptionist screens all EHP calls to determine whether the caller needs to be seen immediately by a clinician:

126

We do some screening and some people say, "Oh, I'm terribly upset, I've got to see somebody right away." "Oh, can you talk a little bit?" "Well, you know, my son doesn't know what medical school to go to and we're just all in a tiz." That can be seen next Tuesday.

Emergencies are relative, as the director pointed out:

Emergency almost always means somebody's anxious. Not necessarily the patient. . . . It could be the supervisor is anxious; the nurse is anxious; a patient. The person is usually doing something that is making somebody else anxious. But whose emergency it is is always up for grabs.

Indeed, this perspective illuminates the program's control mandate. One therapist aptly defined an emergency as

someone who [is] in such severe distress that they need to be seen right away to determine whether they need to be treated or sent out of the workplace because they [are] disruptive to themselves or to the workplace.

Therapists distinguish between true emergencies, which generally require referral to an outside therapist or treatment program, and false emergencies, which can be handled within the program's short-term modalities.

All the staff agree that true emergencies are life-threatening, relatively rare occurrences characterized by someone out of control. One therapist defined a true emergency as involving

some question of possible suicidal tendency. Some question of immediate hospitalization due to a psychotic break. A complete loss of control over behavior. Possible violence to another human being. . . . Those are considered psychiatric emergencies. A threat to the life of the patient or to another person and just the possibility that they might need immediate hospitalization or medication.

The following case related by an intern illustrates several qualities about true emergencies. Others generally identify

127

the employee as being out of control and instigate the employee's referral to the program; the staff members use psychoanalytic terminology to characterize the employee's behavior and loss of control; and the staff members decide to refer the person to an outside resource when their efforts fail to return the employee's behavior to normal.

> I had one . . . that was definitely an emergency. I mean, she flipped out. That was interesting, when we were told we would not see any psychotic patients. . . . [I do not know] whether it was a manic or psychotic or schizo episode, but she definitely had an episode during the workday. She came in in the morning, and she was seen sitting at her desk talking to her typewriter. And no one quite knew what to do. So they just watched it and hoped that it would go away. Then, some of her fellow employees spotted her again in the cafeteria, and she was walking in a circle talking to herself. And they got concerned. And they called the guard to get her up here. And they were able to get her up, and it was quite late in the day. I remember it was about 4:00. We did not get out of here until after 7:00. . . . She was insistent upon going home alone, and we really felt there was no way she could function going into the subway and getting home. And we could not get anybody in—a friend or her mother. And she was incoherent. And we really could not get to her. I mean, one minute she would be perfectly fine, and then we would mention her needing help, and she would disappear. She would disappear. She had been institutionalized at one point, and we finally got hold of the therapist from there and had him talk to her.

False emergencies are characterized as "people who are tearful and who might be overwhelmed at that point in time by a problem." Typically, such distraught employees come to the medical department for help because either they themselves or their supervisor believes that their problem needs immediate attention. Such tearfulness and distress is often interpreted by the nursing staff as an emergency "because the nurse often does not know what to do with such a person" and that impression is communicated to the therapist. What distinguishes a false from a true emergency is that, in a false emergency, the therapist is able to calm the employee and pinpoint a specific problem that has caused the distress and that can be resolved within the short-term modalities. A staff member described a typical false emergency:

> You are in session with someone. There is an eager knock at the door, you answer, and they [the nurses] say, "Hurry up, there's an emergency." So you cancel the session and you are brought into a treatment room and here is a young person crying over the loss of a boyfriend or a girlfriend, let us say. It just happened last night, so they are overwhelmed today. They could not work. You see it also gets translated by the management because the management does not know what to do with someone like this. They then say, "Bring them down to the health center; it's an emergency." They are introduced as an emergency, and it just gets passed along that way.

After a brief discussion of their problem or "a bit of cot rest," employees are often ready to return to work. In instances where the therapist feels that employees are not sufficiently calm to return to work, they are given the remainder of the day off. Many of these employees do not return to the EHP for additional help because they believe either that the crisis has passed or that they are now capable of handling their own problems. Those who do return often feel that the crisis has not yet passed and that they need additional support. Several of the cases demonstrate those characteristics, and are exemplified by Terri A., who was distraught over her marriage, and by Jeannette T., who felt worn out from work and family demands.

Unlike emergency referrals, routine referrals are characterized by calm and order. Indeed, they are routine because employees follow an established procedure: the employee either phones or comes to the medical receptionist to make an appointment and does not communicate that he or she is in crisis. Appointments are typically scheduled within a week of the request. This procedure allows the EHP to control the flow of its work.

Standard routines are characterized as "ideal." Employees involved in standard routines are believed to be "bright," "highly motivated," and "responsive to therapy." Typically, such employees present the therapist with specific problems that they wish to solve (e.g., backaches or a difficult boss) or at least a situation that can be broken down by the therapist into discrete learning objectives. Typically, the employee shows a high level of compliance with the therapist's recommendations and homework assignments.

The following reconstruction of Beverly P.'s case record is a typical example of a standard routine.

First visit The patient is a twenty-six-year-old married, attractive black female of average height and slender build. She arrived for consultation neatly dressed and in a well-groomed manner. She has suffered from temporal-mandibular joint syndrome [TMJ] for five months. ... She is using Valium to alleviate stress and pain but wants to learn to control pain without medication. She is employing a biteplate because of a long-standing braxism.

The patient is alert, and there is no indication of a thought-process disturbance. Her memory is well intact, and she demonstrates good judgment. ...

I recommended that she learn stress-management skills and asked her to keep a daily log of her activities and the onset of pains.

Second visit The patient arrived on time and reported only one mandibular pain problem this week. The patient is actually keeping a daily log. We discussed the onset of her pains, and I encouraged her to continue keeping the log. ... I instructed her in deep-breathing exercises and prescribed that she listen to and follow the instructions on Relaxation Tape no. 3.

Third visit   The patient continues to realize improvement in reducing TMJ and overall pain. The patient is actually listening to, and cooperating with, the relaxation tapes, as well as continuing to perform deep-breathing exercises. . . .

Fourth visit   The patient continues to perform the assigned tasks in a successful manner. The patient reports significantly less TMJ pain and overall stress levels.

Variable routine cases cannot be handled within the program's short-term modality and are, consequently, referred to outside resources. This may occur for any of several reasons: employee requests, alcoholism, or noncompliance.

Many employees request referral to either a private therapist or a treatment agency because they fear a breach of confidentiality if they are treated in the EHP. The therapists always comply with such requests because they recognize employees' concerns about confidentiality as legitimate. There is, however, some tendency to characterize these employees as a bit paranoid:

> You see this concern a great deal with those who have a paranoid personality—the more suspicious and critical types of people. And I think that, regardless of what any program would do, regardless of the reality, that is the perspective that they bring to bear on it and you are not going to make any headway with anyone like that.

While alcoholism cases are also referred to outside treatment because alcoholism treatment generally requires an intensive twenty-eight-day program, it is not always obvious in the intake interview that an employee has a drinking problem. One therapist commented that

> alcoholism, for example, often does not emerge immediately, and it becomes the primary diagnosis when you

realize that that was the problem. Because of the massive denial, very often they con the therapist beautifully. You are off on the wrong tangent for a while until you begin to get the feeling that that is where it is at.

Once such a diagnosis is made, the therapist encourages the employee to go to a rehabilitation program.

It can also be difficult to identify noncompliant employees in the intake interview. But once they are identified on the basis of their unwillingness to work on their problems and do homework assignments, they are encouraged either to work on their problems or to seek additional help from outside resources. Such clients are sometimes described as "psychology-wise." "They know all the jargon. They have read all the books," and, as one therapist stated,

> Our responsibility is to cut those people off or make the appropriate recommendations. . . . They are not consciously malingering. They really do need help but have not yet been able to accept that fact—but in their apparent, earnest desire to get help are really avoiding it. They are hard to get to.

The noncompliant client, however, is not typical of the program's clientele, and reports of significant improvement were fairly common in the case records of the employees interviewed. Consequently, it is not too surprising that the therapists say that working in the program is a satisfying experience.

> You can make an impact on these people. You rarely find a situation where you have that constant futility that many psychologists feel from their patient load. When these folks come here, you can actually see improvement through biofeedback and cognitive-behavioral interventions.

Limitations on treatment

The EHP's preference for short-term cognitive-behavioral therapy is limited not only by Corpco's economics and by the

132

therapists' professional training. It is also a political decision designed to satisfy the demands made upon the program by both the employees and the organization and to deal with the necessity of maintaining the program as an ongoing entity.

When employees come to the EHP, they seek an answer to their problems; however, they will not accept just any answer. Many will not accept medication, nor will they accept the more painful and coercive forms of behavior modification (e.g., aversive conditioning), which have been discredited by such critics as Peter Schrag (1978) and Robert Geiser (1976). Indeed, these forms of treatment have generally been used on such powerless subjects as patients confined to mental institutions and criminals incarcerated in prisons. In contrast, Corpco employees are free either to use or not to use the EHP services. So in order to assure themselves of a clientele, the therapists rely upon the more benign forms of behavioral therapy (e.g., biofeedback) and stress the program's voluntary nature and the employees' responsibility in the continuance of treatment. As one therapist aptly expresses it, "They are a partner and indeed the prime mover in the process of symptom relief."

Employee preferences also limit the therapists' discretion in making outside referrals. This is dramatically evident with true emergencies. In such cases therapists often interpret an employee's behavior as requiring immediate hospitalization. When the employee refuses such a recommendation, commitment procedures (Zusman 1976) make it difficult for the therapist to do more than encourage him or her to do so. The following report from a staff member illustrates this limitation:

> She started to talk about suicide. And I had not seen her for quite a long time, and I really sensed something very different in the way she was talking that day. . . . We wanted to get her into Roosevelt Hospital, and we could not force her to go. We were ready, [another therapist] and I, to get into a cab with her and drag her into the hospital for what we felt was her own good. But, never-

133

theless, you cannot do that. So we let her go. . . . [We] went out with our fingers crossed, just hoping she would get home.

Beyond the requirement that the EHP deliver cost-effective services, Corpco makes an even more basic demand: the EHP may not disrupt the workplace or disturb the status quo. Infractions of this requirement can result in the firing of therapists and even in program termination. This limitation affects the length of treatment and the therapists' use of group therapy and of structural change as possible intervention strategies.

The question of treatment length is not only a question of what is cost-effective. It is also a question of how much time Corpco will tolerate an employee's being away from his or her desk, and it appears that some managers had been pressed to the limits of their tolerance. The current director stated this several times during my research, and, as one therapist pointed out, "A lot of them [employees] were in trouble on the job. And then having to leave the job for an hour, once a week, sometimes twice a week, I do not think endeared them to their supervisors. It was just one more thing."

Group therapy is a standard treatment option in psychologists' private practices. While management has never discouraged its use in the EHP, the logistics of assembling a group of people during the workday are extremely difficult.

> The major disadvantage in working in a corporate setting is you are working only . . . with the client. In private practice, you have the luxury of pulling in the extended family and whomever else is involved in the primary problem. If the son comes, for example, the whole family can be involved working with the problem. . . . The logistics [in a corporate setting] make it virtually impossible.

In spite of these difficulties, two therapists did report working with family groups, and one intern was able to conduct a six-week stress-management workshop for fifty employees by using two lunch hours a week.

Current mental health literature extolls the effectiveness of support groups in helping individuals to cope with stressful situations (e.g., Turner 1981, Williams et al. 1981). The former director said, "The single most effective form of stress management is social support. And you cannot ever forget that. And you have got to provide more opportunities for that." To a startling degree, Corpco has done just that by encouraging employees to participate in such groups as its People's Network and its Rotating Advisory Panels (RAPs). The company developed both groups to help employees cope more effectively with work-related problems. Nevertheless, as one woman's description of her People's Network group attests, the groups also function to defuse potential conflict between management and workers.

> We meet every other week. We have been meeting now for two years. We can discuss any problem that we have. . . . Mostly work issues. Things in the office. Things that you want to cope with. . . . We are very discreet about who we get. . . . We do not want somebody who is derogatory toward the company. In other words, this is not a people's group where you knock the company. They are there to build ourselves up and what we should do to further our own goals.

The three RAPs are advisory groups to the president that focus on minority issues of concern to women, blacks, and hispanics. Each group is composed of six people who serve for one year. Typically, individuals in these groups develop close relationships and continue to meet with one another after their tenure expires.

> You really have to meet with the president every two months. . . . And you have to bring up topics for discussion. It is a real personal growth experience because you cannot say anything negative. On the other hand, you are not there just to pat him on the back. So you are trying to accomplish something in a good, positive way.

There is a limit to what management will tolerate in a support group. That limit is reached when employees say derogatory things about the company and when they begin to organize independently. Corpco swiftly punishes such behavior. This was dramatically demonstrated when the cleaning staff attempted to unionize. A therapist explained:

> I had strong feelings about the way the company handled its cleaning staff. . . . They were fired because they were disgruntled. They felt their benefits and their salaries were not in keeping with other employees in the company, and, therefore, they began to be interested in union people who came around. . . . Corpco, which has never had a union shop, fired everybody. . . . What they did was they fired all these people, and they said, "But don't worry. You'll still be working here. The building still has to get clean. What we are doing is, we are going to hire a consulting company that only does cleaning for industry. And that company has promised that they are going to hire all of you and that your job will be the same you have now, only all your pay and your benefits will come from them. . . ." It was true. The firm that was brought in to do the cleaning kept those people for several weeks—and then they fired 70 percent.

Corpco discourages structural changes that disturb the status quo. Although the therapists focus on the individual, they are well aware that many of the employees' problems stem from the way work is organized and that, in instances where the majority of employees in one area report similar stress reactions, there is a likelihood of ineffective management practices that need to be changed. With this in mind, the former director developed a "stress barometer" to identify such areas. But the technique never advanced from the conceptual stage because of management fears that such an instrument would be disruptive. Indeed, the EHP has been told that organizational change is not its task and that when employees have legitimate work problems they should be handled by the established procedure.

The established procedure refers an employee with work complaints to either Echo Voice, which is the company's arbitration system, or to the Equal Employment Opportunities officer. Links between these programs and the EHP are tenuous at best. The EHP staff had sketchy knowledge about them, and one of the staff volunteered, "These areas have a reputation for not maintaining confidentiality . . . so most people did not go there." The current director is attempting to strengthen the relationship between Echo Voice and the EHP, but he admits that the interns seem to have the impression that Echo Voice is a "sop" and that the employees referred there "would be placated and made to feel like a bad person if they could not get along in the wonderful company." The only remaining option for therapists concerned about problems in the workplace is to recommend that the company undertake human relations training to teach managers good supervisory practices.

My interviews revealed a variety of limitations on the therapists' work. What happens when therapists exceed those limits? The simple truth appears to be that the therapists are terminated. Before my arrival at Corpco, a full-time salaried psychologist was either fired or forced to resign. It is difficult to know which actually did occur, because I was not present and the staff were reluctant to talk about it. Nevertheless, I can say that the psychologist's departure clearly defined for the staff the consequences of exceeding their boundaries (Erikson 1966). The departed psychologist was described as an "employee advocate," who refused to keep case records in the medical files because she did not believe those files were really confidential and who habitually saw patients beyond the allotted time. Upon her departure, it was rumored that she was suing Corpco for forcing her to abandon her patients. One therapist commented on the ambivalence that most of the staff felt about this situation.

It was unclear if she [the psychologist] was being fired or if she was resigning or who was at fault. Well, to a large degree, all of that was kept private and away from the interns. . . . [We were] aware of bits and pieces of information without knowing the whole story. And there were times at which that became difficult because of the political nature of the place. . . . But there were times when she tried to pull me into things that were going on with her. And it was tricky because she was a person too. She had a point of view, and some of her beefs were legitimate too.

Treating employees

Cognitive-behavioral therapy is currently fashionable among psychologists, and the *Annual Review of Behavior Therapy* designated 1976 as the Year of Cognition (Wilson 1980). Some of its most important contributors (Beck 1976, Ellis and Grieger 1977, and Meichenbaum 1977) view the current fascination with cognitive factors in therapy as the means of facilitating a long-awaited integration of the traditional psychodynamic approach with behavior therapy. Cognitive-behavioral therapy is rooted in social learning theory, exemplified by Albert Bandura's work (1969, 1977). Bandura emphasizes the importance of thought processes in regulating individual behavior and rejects the unidirectional causal models of psychoanalysis, which emphasizes autonomous psychic forces, and of radical behaviorism, which emphasizes strict operant conditioning. Rather, Bandura's reciprocal determinism model depicts psychological functioning as involving a continuous interdependence of individual behavior, thought processes, and external events. According to this model, individuals are seen as being acted upon by their environment and reacting to that environment according to the manner in which they see the world.

138

Central to all the cognitive-behavioral therapies is the notion that stress is a normal part of the environment and that healthy individuals develop skills that allow them to cope adequately with their environment (Davidson and Davidson 1980). Cognitive-behavioral therapists define stress as an "unfavorable perception of the social environment and its dynamics" (Brown 1980, 90). Stress is "manufactured by the mind" when an individual interprets a social situation as unfavorable to his or her well-being because he or she cannot understand, accept, or rationalize that situation. It is a problem to be solved and is analogous to what is commonly called worrying. The inability to find an acceptable solution to a problem causes one to worry more, and this in turn can result in an inability to function socially or in one of the stress-related illnesses. The function of therapy is to increase the kind and amount of information a person has, so that the individual can solve the problem. Such an increase may come from simply gathering more information about one's situation or from perceiving the situation in a new light.

The cognitive-behavioral therapy of the EHP is based on this notion of increasing information in order to increase employees' options for understanding and solving their problems, and as the former director explained, the responsibility for using that information belongs to the employee.

> The clients should play a very, very active role, because it is their problem, and they are the ones that have got to do something about it. So that your orientation should be toward getting the client involved, engaged in prescriptive exercises, which are based on sound behavioral modification and cognitive alteration principles. And that you serve as a teacher, as an educator, for the client, and that education is aimed at coping better and alleviating the symptoms and changing adverse life situations rather than listening to the pain again and again and again. . . . That is the basis for our belief in the whole array of basically self-regulatory types of approaches that we em-

139

ploy. The ultimate responsibility is the patient's, and what we will do is work with them in order to make them better at managing their lives, at coping with the problems of living, at getting rid of symptoms.

The program uses a number of techniques in order to increase the information that employees have about themselves and their behavior: keeping daily activity logs, hypnosis, relaxation tapes, and biofeedback.

Biofeedback is the most frequently used tool in the program, and it is usually used to help individuals cope with stress-related physiological symptoms. Biofeedback gives employees a graphic image of their physiological processes and requires them to spend a great deal of time focusing upon their internal dynamics. It allows therapists to teach employees how to cope with their problems and encourages employees to take responsibility for those problems.

For the better part of a century, psychophysiologists have been using instruments to measure and record changes in heart rate, blood pressure, blood flow, respiration, muscle tension, and brain waves in response to changes in thoughts and emotions. It was the accident of turning those instruments around to face the people being recorded that revealed the biofeedback phenomenon (Brown 1980). The biofeedback instrument senses body signals that individuals cannot or do not consciously perceive, and converts these signals into forms that can be perceived quite easily (e.g., flashing lights, noise, and numerical displays). These signals represent certain physiological changes and are used by the individual to become acquainted with internal events, especially since the instruments are designed to follow the dynamic activity of the physiology as it varies over time. The biofeedback phenomenon is what happens when people have the opportunity to spend time observing the ongoing changes in their own internal states and when they are instructed in how to change the physiological functions. They learn that they can develop full voluntary control over selected physical functions. The means used to produce the changes are chiefly mental, such as imagining relaxation or using self-suggestion to change the physiological functions or shifting consciousness to a passive state.

Learning biofeedback is a novel experience for employees in which they are hooked up to the machine and able to receive accurate information about their physiological functioning. The therapists help the employees adjust to the situation by being friendly and telling them that anyone can learn to change body activities within the first hour of treatment.

The EHP therapists give biofeedback generally high marks.

> The main value of the biofeedback technique is that it really shows people visually and strongly that they can have an effect on their bodies. That they really can use their intellect to determine the way they respond in certain situations. And I think that is important for people to realize. And I do not know if saying it to somebody is as effective as them seeing that red, green, yellow light flashing on and off.

The employees themselves are enthusiastic about biofeedback. Mary Margaret O. came to the EHP about her migraines, and her enthusiasm after two sessions was fairly typical.

> It is really amazing because [the therapist] said that my levels were like the highest she has seen in people that she has dealt with. Like the highest is 20 something, and I got down the other day to a 4 something. I'm really working at it. I'm [also] listening to the relaxation tapes.

"Working at it" is one of the major ways in which employees learn to take responsibility for their problems. This means following the therapists' instructions about keeping the daily log, listening to the relaxation tapes, or doing deep-breathing exercises. Mary Margaret spends a considerable amount of time each day working at it:

> Every night without fail I do it for a half-hour or 45 minutes. . . . I have to push myself to do it in the morn-

ing. . . . I have been trying to get up a little earlier. So, like yesterday, I did it for 10 minutes and, then, when I came in for the session, I started at a lower count than I did last time.

Working at it and seeing tangible results help convince employees that they are responsible.

Biofeedback is used in conjunction with cognitive psychotherapy. As the therapists are quick to point out,

> Biofeedback can be an extremely effective technique— but used in the hands of a trained therapist, not in the hands of an untrained therapist or a technician. Research has shown just a biofeedback technician has very little effect on a patient's symptomology. They have been doing a study in California using biofeedback technicians versus a psychotherapist where psychotherapy also was given before and after the actual biofeedback session. Only in that condition were there positive gains for the patient.

Indeed, once employees learn that they can control their body, they are encouraged to transfer this learning to the control of their environment. Cognitive psychotherapy encourages them to believe that many of the problems that they encounter and that cause them to be stressed are a function of the way they see and react to the world. Biofeedback makes them realize they can change their physical reactions, and cognitive psychotherapy makes them realize they can change their mental reactions.

In Mary Margaret O.'s case, psychotherapy consisted of discussing the unreasonable demands that she makes upon herself.

> I [am] too hard on myself. That is why I have all these pressure signs coming out of my head on the machine.

At the time I interviewed her, she was holding down a full-time, demanding job, helping to pay for a new house, trying to become pregnant, and trying to keep up relations with her own and her husband's very large families. With the help of her therapist she was beginning to sort out which of those activities had high and low priorities and to develop new coping strategies. Her therapist said Mary Margaret was "a good candidate for biofeedback and motivated to enter treatment."

When employees come to the program seeking help with marital or family problems, the therapists use cognitive psychotherapy in order to increase the amount of information employees have about their situation and in order to help them see their problems from a new perspective. Ideally, such information and perception should help them develop new coping strategies. Management considers such problems safe because they are typically short-term crises that are solvable, do not cause major disruptions in the workplace, and do not raise questions about how work is organized. The current director said these are the kinds of cases that the company likes the EHP to handle. The program enables these employees to manage their own resources, and, at the same time, it enables them to stay at work and function productively. These cases benefit the company's employee relations because these employees generally feel that the company has done something for them.

When asked what technique they would use in the case of Terri A., whose husband had left her, all the staff members stated that they would use some form of cognitive psychotherapy.

> Well, I would let her cry. And I would try to help her see in what ways she can survive—first of all, that she *will* survive—and what she can do that will make surviving easier for her. I would try to really get more on a rational-emotive form of therapy. . . . see the bottom line—what the fear is, what would happen to her, now that he has left—to get her feelings on his leaving. The marriage was not happy. . . . He does not want it; he wants out. . . . But I think the immediate thing would

be just to get her to see what her fears are and if there really is any kind of rational basis for them.

Terri A.'s case record corroborates this.

First visit   The patient is coping with the entire blame for her marriage break-up. She knows this is wrong on an intellectual level but cannot resolve her real role in the marriage failure. Although she is attractive, she has a poor self-image. She wants her husband back even though she states the marriage was bad from the beginning. The husband's family rejected her, and the husband seemed unable or unwilling to build a depth relationship.

Second visit   The patient continues to dwell on the past. She reports depression and sleep disturbances. Through the use of focused restructuring, she is beginning to conclude that her needs were not met, and possibly could not be met, by her former husband. She wants to concentrate on the present and near future. She recognizes that she is not alone and can learn a lesson from this experience.

Third visit   The patient had a brief contact with her husband which brought on feelings of anger and depression. She has decided that further contact would serve no positive purpose. Increasingly, she is able to concentrate on and to plan activities for herself with positive outcomes. She is involved in social activities with female friends. . . . She is less disturbed, able to laugh and smile, and better able to focus on the positive in the present.

. . . .

Sixth visit   The patient has planned a number of activities and feels better. She considers all men "snakes in the grass" and exhibits hostility whenever discussing men. Her anger is apparent, and we discussed this, particularly her selective perspective of their behavior to reinforce her basic assumption. This means she has to discount or distort contrary information. This makes it impossible for her to have a meaningful relationship, which she claims that she wants. Also by blaming men, she absolves herself, and this gives her license to treat them badly. This had never been put to her this way before, and she, I believe, is beginning to recognize and want change.

Terri admitted that when she came to the program her perspective was distorted.

> I was ashamed to say anything, which is something [the therapist] has helped me to overcome. . . . There was about a week after I had seen [the therapist] where I would not even go outside of the house. I was terrified. I thought everybody knows. "You did it; it is all your fault. . . ." I wouldn't even go to the candy store. . . . Finally, [the therapist] told me this cannot continue.

It has not. Her homework (e.g., keeping her daily log, reading prescribed articles) and her discussions with the therapist, have enabled Terri to see new hope for herself, and she is rebuilding her world.

Cognitive therapy is also used to treat employees who come to the program because of work problems and stress-related illnesses. Many of them are put on the biofeedback machine and taught relaxation techniques. Essentially, the therapists use two strategies with these employees: they attempt to teach employees how to cope better with their present position and boss, and when the first strategy does not work, they attempt to make employees see that they are in the wrong job and should seek another.

One therapist explained the first strategy:

> We can help [the employee] to cope better with his supervisor and also to learn strategies to turn situations around to get the supervisor to be less of a problem, less of a stress-carrier. And that makes the patient more com-

145

petent and masterful in those situations. . . . [When] the patient learns to cope better, he or she [the supervisor] becomes less overwhelming, less awesome, brought down to size. . . . The person loses their highly charged negative characteristics when the person sees that the patient is coping. They are not as nearly so difficult to handle. I would say that [is true] in 99 percent of the cases.

When employees cannot learn to cope with their boss or position, the therapists encourage them to seek alternative employment. This strategy is based on contingency management theory, which suggests that there are appropriate and inappropriate matches of employees with certain personality types and work environments with certain characteristics (Harrison 1978). The theory of person-environment fit was expressed succinctly by one of the therapists:

In a lot of cases, this is not the right fit for a person, and to try and adapt to this company would be detrimental to the person. As I said, they [the employees] are our primary responsibility. I have told people, "Get the hell out of here. This isn't the right spot for you." And I would not have any trouble defending that to the company, because why would the company want misfit sorts of employees who are not going to produce and are miserable. I mean, there are plenty of other people to fill that position that might be just perfect for the job.

Mary M. came to the program because of her conflict with an aggressive M.B.A. and because she felt her supervisor was discriminating against her. The reconstruction of her case record illustrates the alternative employment strategy.

First visit   The patient has a "workplace problem." She is very angry and disappointed about her job. She feels her boss has not fulfilled his promises to her. . . . She feels her manager cannot relate to women well. She copes with mistreatment by acceptance. Her anxiety is the result of frustration and outrage at being thwarted.

She tried talking to her coworker (MBA), but he closed off altogether. . . . Her frustration level is high. I prescribed Dalmane to help her sleep.

Second visit   The patient reports a hangover from Dalmane and says she is falling asleep all day. She napped 2 hours on Saturday and is "catching up" on sleep.

Third visit   The patient wants to put money to the injustice she feels. I pointed out that she should have only one goal, which is to be successful. She says she wants (a) more responsibility and advancement, (b) justice, and (c) revenge. She got angry when I suggested that if (a) was her real goal she should transfer to another department or to another company. She has already planned to do this. It is very sad about that reality. If she is right her boss does not want her to do much.

Mary said of her encounter with the therapist,

I think sometimes talking to a counselor, a psychologist, does not solve the problem but gives you comfort. I can let it out, and I know that somebody is listening to me. I think that is about it. . . . I am seeing a solution to the problem. The solution is to leave the job.

She left and found a better job. Her therapist reported,

I do have a letter from [Mary]. . . . She was bitching and moaning that she was not respected enough and that she was not getting paid enough and went to see a career counselor and found out she could double her money based on her skills and experience and her credentials. And it had nothing to do with being a woman or whatever, etc.; it had something to do with the position she had was not paying enough and she had a lot more talent and skills.

Mary's case ended happily for all parties. She found a better-paying job, the company avoided a discrimination suit, and the therapist felt good about his recommendation. But what about those employees who are deflected to other employers but have fewer skills, less experience, and fewer credentials than Mary? One therapist answered,

> [Some people] do not have a lot of alternatives on the outside. I mean, some people, they need this job desperately. The lower-grade employees, they do not want to lose their job, but they are having so much difficulty coping that they are going to. So those folks we definitely want to help adapt to the organization.

Medical diagnosis and treatment are socially constructed artifacts rather than scientific accomplishments. Both occur within the context of management requirements, professional beliefs, and employee demands. Corpco management requires that the EHP deliver cost-effective services without disrupting the workplace and that all organization-employee conflicts be resolved in its favor. The EHP psychologists believe that employee concerns can be traced to the individual's inability to cope and that cognitive-behavioral therapy is the most appropriate treatment for such problems. Employees demand answers to their problems and reject medication and aversive forms of behavioral modification.

From these limitations emerge actual diagnoses and treatments. They are socially constructed artifacts. Diagnosis functions principally as a professional justification to Corpco's management and employees rather than as a guideline for choosing an appropriate treatment. In fact, treatment decisions are based upon simplified processing stereotypes rather than upon scientifically derived diagnoses, and these stereotypes result from the EHP's desire to satisfy management's requirement for short-term therapy and its own need to control its work by selecting "good" treatment candidates.

While EHP therapists experience a great deal of autonomy in creating diagnoses and treating employees, their contention that this allows them to resolve all company-worker conflicts in the employee's favor does not ring true. As illustrated in several episodes in this chapter, social control is intrinsic to the EHP therapists' role. It is apparent in their reaction to employees who enter the program as emergency referrals. They physically isolate employees displaying disruptive behavior from their coworkers and do not allow them to return to their work areas until the therapists confirm that they are no longer out of control. It is also apparent in the handling of routine referrals, in which instances the therapists perceive themselves as helping employees to resolve their problems before they get out of hand and disrupt either their families or work lives.

The social control aspect of the therapists' role is emphasized by their commitment to cognitive-behavioral therapy and Corpco's restrictions on the use of group therapies and structural changes. These strictures virtually assure that employees seek individualized solutions to their problems and eschew group-based ones. Although individualized solutions may be appropriate for such personal decisions as whether to return to one's spouse, they are not always the most appropriate ones for solving work-related issues, which may require changes in the status quo. When therapists encourage individual solutions to work-related problems and discourage group-based ones that challenge the status quo, they resolve such conflicts in the company's favor and help to ensure that work continues to be done according to management's directives.

Indeed, when EHP therapists pursue person-environment fit strategies with employees, they demonstrate how closely their treatment ideology parallels management theory and betray an absence of therapeutic neutrality. Like their military counterparts, the EHP therapists have made a successful bureaucratic adaptation by incorporating Corpco's business rationale into their treatment ideology, which allows them to go about their work without feeling that they are captives of the organization.

6. Social consequences

Focusing on the social ramifications of defining troubles as a medical problem, this chapter examines the consequences for the employees, management, and the program staff of using the emotional health program. These consequences inhere in medicalization itself and occur regardless of the validity of medical diagnoses or the effectiveness of medical treatment.

Peter Conrad and Joseph Schneider (1980a) discuss both the "brighter" and "darker" sides of defining troubles as medical problems in society. The social benefits include the creation of humanitarian and nonpunitive sanctions; the extension of the sick role to some troublesome individuals; a reduction of individual responsibility, blame, and possibly stigma; an optimistic therapeutic ideology; care and treatment rendered by a prestigious profession; and the availability of a more flexible and often more efficient means of social control. The darker consequences of medicalization include the dislocation of responsibility, the assumption of the moral neutrality of medicine, domination by expert control, medical social control, the individualization of social problems, the depoliticization of troublesome behavior, and the exclusion of evil. The social ramifications of using the EHP parallel these brighter and darker consequences.

150

Consequences for employees

Employees who refer themselves to the EHP experience two social consequences. First, they feel stigmatized by their involvement in the program, and this perception prompts them to conceal their involvement from others. Second, by complying with the psychotherapists' instructions, they experience a secondary gain that allows them to recontain their problems within the contexts of their family and work lives.

Historically, practitioners have contended that defining troublesome conditions and behaviors as medical problems reduces the stigma associated with them; however, little empirical evidence exists to substantiate this claim (Conrad and Schneider 1980a). Indeed, Derek Phillips' (1963) research suggests that people seeking medical advice for their personal problems heavily risk being rejected and stigmatized, and the more recent surveys of Veroff and his colleagues (1981) suggest that many people continue to resist going to psychotherapy because of what others will think. Employees who refer themselves to the EHP fear that others will reject them if their involvement is discovered.

Employees come to the EHP to learn to contain the signs and symptoms of what they perceive to be a discreditable attribute and, ironically, program involvement induces its own stigma, against which they must guard themselves further. The fear of being discredited because of their EHP involvement is expressed in several ways. First, as one therapist explained, they avoid acknowledging the EHP staff when they encounter the staff outside the EHP offices.

> Even though the confidentiality is not breached, [it is] always in the back of your head. "I wonder if anyone will ever know?" Outside of this setting, like in the cafeteria, when other people see me, patients, many of them will look away and avoid me because there is somebody else in this building that knows personal and private things about [them]. I think that gives them pause, and I think it should.

Employees also express this fear directly. Ann Z., speaking about her coworkers' finding out that she has been seeing a Corpco psychotherapist, said,

> People think, because you are asking for help, you are weak and there is something wrong with you. Even though in this day and age everyone has an analyst or something like that. . . . It is so gossipy on the floor, and the minute something is known the whole world [knows]. I mean, I really do not care what kind of gossip they talk, I just do not want to be it.

Beverly P. feared that, if her coworkers knew, they would not understand:

> If they understood why I came here [the EHP], it would not bother me, but I do not think they could understand why I came here. They would go, "Ah, she's crazy!" That is the first thing that goes through their minds. Crazy! Like, [my friend], she really understands that I am coming here because of my mouth, and maybe I can get some kind of control [over my TMJ pain]. It is not really a mental problem. . . . Not many people will understand it really. Understand that your face can hurt. They would not believe it; so I won't discuss it with them.

Concealment of one's involvement in the EHP is only partial, as Kevin D. reported, because employees engage in selective telling.

> I am very careful who I mention this [biofeedback treatment] to because people can take things the wrong way. . . . I do not think I would bring it up as a matter of conversation at lunch. "Oh, by the way fellows." It is really nobody's business other than my own family.

Although Kevin believed that his treatment is only his family's concern, Patricia O. planned to keep her biofeedback treatment secret from her mother.

I am careful who I tell about it. My own family does not know yet. My mother, of course her reaction would be, "You're getting like your sister!" So I would not tell her about it.

In order to manage the stigma potential of visiting the EHP, employees selectively tell trusted others about their involvement in order to elicit assurances that they are not crazy and that the EHP services can be beneficial. Ellen S. needed such assurances:

[My girlfriend] thought it was super. She said I should not be embarrassed about it or anything. For the first two or three times that I went [to the EHP], it was like I am holding this in [and] I got to tell somebody about it. So I told my aunt, and I told my girlfriend. Now it is so much easier for me. . . . It is just a so much more relaxing atmosphere for her [the aunt] to know that I am not doing it on the sneak, that I am involved with it, and that she just accepted it.

Terri A.'s statement suggests how selectively telling others elicits encouragement for employees to continue with the EHP because they believe it is helpful:

I have two coworkers that I am real close to. They know. My family knows. . . . [They were] real glad that I went. That was a sign that Terri does want to help herself. And I did.

Employees also tell others whom they believe can benefit from the EHP service, although others were not always quick to accept such suggestions. Mary Margaret O. encouraged a coworker to refer herself to the EHP.

She [the coworker] wants to go [to biofeedback] for stress. She gets very depressed, and if things really bother her, she cries really easily. . . . I keep pushing her because now I know it is helping me. So I keep pushing her. I keep telling her to make an appointment.

153

Mary M., who came because of her conflict with the young M.B.A., told a coworker and received a cool response.

> I told one of the other girls because she is very, very upset. She said, "I'm gonna take that guy [the M.B.A.] and break his face." She came to my office. I told her that she should go down to the [EHP] because it is not just you and I that are upset. It is everyone in the area here. I feel that someone should know about this because it is poor management. . . . She did not say too much, but I did not think she was willing to come. . . . She does not believe in counseling. See, a lot of people are turned off by anything to do with psychology. They say, "I'm not crazy!"

Again and again employees stated that they believed that others equated seeing a psychologist with being crazy. Not surprisingly, even though they are very selective in choosing whom they tell about their involvement and usually receive support and encouragement, on occasion employees receive an adverse response from someone. As Terri A. recounted, these responses further reinforce the awareness of stigma attached to using the EHP.

> There are a few friends that I had told because I am not ashamed of it. . . . There were two people who said, "Hey, are you nuts?" "No, I'm not nuts. How dare you say that?" . . . I got angry. . . . They did not understand at all. [It was] ignorance on their part. . . . [They] took me by surprise. I did not think that they were so closed-minded about speaking to a psychologist or a psychoanalyst.

Employees worry about the permanence of their emotional health records and about what would happen if those diagnoses fell into someone else's hands. Lorraine P. was clearly concerned about this possibility.

> I had an aunt who was a school principal. One of the kids got pulled in by the truant officer. . . . [the student]

quietly said [to my aunt], "Sister, does this mean I have a police record?" And she [the aunt] said, "I wanted to tell her 'yes' to impress her, but I was afraid that she would get picked up for a traffic violation and would get asked that question and [that she would] say 'yes' and get in all sorts of trouble. So I said to her, 'Well, I don't think the first offense you do.' " I thought of that. . . . I wonder if this is on my record, that I am emotionally unstable. How can I explain that if it ever showed up anywhere? I suppose it is not totally sensible, because I certainly would not object to anyone knowing that I had gone through a biofeedback training series for relaxation. That would not bother me. But to have been in the Emotional Health Program, I would want to keep that quiet.

Indeed, all of the employees hope that their EHP involvement will be kept quiet, and like Ann Z. they all accept that there is some risk involved.

I am pretty sure everything is confidential. . . . [If] as I work and I do not get the promotions I feel I should get and the reasons do not sound rational, that means they must be holding it against me. . . . But I do not get the feeling that it is going to be anything like that. At least I am hoping. . . .

The employees' visits to the EHP are recorded in two places: in the psychiatric files and in the computer. The computer record is abbreviated and consists of the individual's employee number, the date of his or her visit to the EHP, the code number of the therapist who treated the employee, and one of four general diagnoses: schizophrenic disorder, neurotic disorder, substance abuse, and other mental disorder. Theoretically, this computer record is used to audit the EHP's activities, and it is accessible only to those individuals who possess the correct computer code, such as the medical and emotional health program directors, their business administrators, and Corpco's auditors. While employees know that

Corpco keeps the psychiatric file, I do not know how aware they are of the computer file.

While the program staff makes every effort to maintain confidentiality, accidents do happen, and information can leak out of the files. In fact, in one mysterious incident, described by the director, the computer printed out an employee's diagnosis and had it sent to the employee.

> Somehow a form got into the computer on a guy that I put down [as] "possible paranoid schizophrenia." And, [I do not know] how the hell this document got into the computer and got sent back to him! . . . He came in terrified—"What does this mean?"

The mystery remains. Fortunately, this particular diagnosis was sent to the employee himself. But one need only ask what might have happened had the diagnosis been sent to a prospective boss to envision the permanence of the attached label and its attendant consequences. Indeed, at present there is no real assurance that the label "possible paranoid schizophrenic" will not appear on someone's video display terminal twenty or thirty years from now.

By complying with the therapists' recommendations, employees reduce stress on themselves and learn to cope more effectively with their problems. These results enable the employees to recontain their problems within the context of their family and work lives. Recontainment, is a secondary gain that follows from the employee's assumption of the sick role (Parsons 1951), whereby he or she is exempted from some obligations in return for recognizing that the problem is undesirable and cooperating with the therapist.

In order to take advantage of the gain from the sick role, employees must engage in instrumental telling. They tell family members, managers, or coworkers of their involvement in the EHP in order to gain release from some obligations.

Ruth B. came to the EHP complaining that her hearing and vision were impaired. She characterized herself as a very nervous person and attributed the onset of her physical problems to the unreasonable demands made upon her by her family. By complying with the EHP therapist's recommendations, she was able to secure release from her family obligations.

> Ever since . . . I came to Medical and started seeing Dr. Whyte, my weekends have not been as hectic because I will not let them be hectic. I told myself that I am not going to run around for everybody. Then I do not accomplish anything. So I have slowed down a lot. . . . You see, I was like the only driver in this family, and I always do all the driving for everybody: my mother, my niece, my nephew. If they have to go somewhere, I have to go somewhere. I have to wait for them. I have to pick them up. And it used to aggravate me. . . . I just do not do it anymore.

Jeanette T. came to the EHP when she found that work and family demands were restricting the time that she had to socialize with her friends. Again, by complying with the therapist's recommendations, she was now able to secure release from some of her household chores.

> This [keeping the daily activity log] is the one thing that has helped. . . . By marking down the different types of stress on the chart they give you, you realize that what adds up is when you have another bathroom to clean and a thing to vacuum, and you want to go to the pool with your friends. I said, "Look at how this thing [the graph] is going up. I'm rushing. Phooey! I'm going to put on my bathing suit; I'm going out with my friends." I stayed there 3–4 hours, and the next day, I went to my other friend's pool. It is a wonderful thing to see in black and white.

In Jeanette T.'s case, EHP involvement also helped her to regain control of her work life. When she told her managers about the stress engendered by the work situation and her subsequent involvement with biofeedback, they agreed to give her additional help with her tasks.

> I came back and mentioned [the visit to the EHP] to them. They were concerned. If I, who thrive on this [busy schedule], am having trouble, [then what]? Since then . . . we are getting an additional person. . . . There is a lot of work involved with . . . the job to bring it up to fit this person. I am getting her, and I am getting another person to help with the running of the office. So even though we will have the same pace, we will have the support that a leader should have. So that if we want to take a vacation, we can.

Patricia O., who attributed her choking partly to the unreasonable demands of her alcoholic boss, was able to get him to stop screaming at her after she told him about her stress reaction to his unreasonableness and her subsequent EHP involvement.

> Since I have told him [about the choking and biofeedback treatment], I have noticed he does not scream at me anymore. I guess I got to him some way. He must have gone home and thought about it. He stopped screaming.

For many employees merely being away from the office for an hour was helpful in dealing with work. One therapist believed that

> sometimes one of the most therapeutic parts of that system was that people got away from a horrible work situation for an hour a week. Especially, if their supervisor was a really destructive person or something.

While those employees who do comply with the therapist's recommendations often are able to regain control of their family and work lives, failure to comply with the therapist's instructions can result in a complete breakdown of these relationships.

In Salvatore I.'s case, noncompliance led to the loss of his job. Salvatore came to the EHP at the insistence of his supervisor, who was concerned about his declining job performance and drinking behavior. Salvatore disagreed with his supervisor's evaluation of his problem. He insisted that his work was declining because he was bored with doing the same job day in and day out, and he believed that he needed career counseling, not alcoholism treatment. The therapist worked with him for three months. She did career and marital counseling with him while continuing to encourage him to attend Alcoholics Anonymous. Although he attended two or three AA meetings, he continued to insist that he did not have a drinking problem and that everything would be all right if he got a new job. Finally, his supervisor notified the therapist that she was placing Salvatore on probation because his lunch hour drinking rendered him nonfunctional in the afternoon and because he was focusing on work that was not relevant to his job. Salvatore continued to drink. His job performance did not improve, and six weeks after being put on probation, he was fired.

Consequences for management

There are three consequences of EHP use that directly benefit Corpco's management. First, the program allows employees to glimpse the human side of enterprise, and, if one believes the human relations theorists (e.g., McGregor 1960), this increases employee morale and commitment to the company. Second, EHP use reinforces the process of the individualization of social problems, and, third, it encourages the depoliticization of the workplace.

Medicalization is related to a long-term humanitarian trend in the conception and control of trouble (Conrad and Schneider 1980a). Indeed, medicine and humanitarianism developed concurrently, and medical definitions of problems are considered the scientific and humane way of viewing a problem. Corpco's EHP is an expression of these sentiments. It allows management to express a personal concern for employees' problems and to suggest that they regard the employee as

159

something more than a cog in the production process. As the EHP director said, "From upper management's point of view, there is an idealistic, humanitarian venture involved [in the EHP]." The therapists agree that managers perceive the program as a means of reaching out to employees and demonstrating concern for them as individuals.

> [Supervisors refer employees to the EHP] because they are concerned about [work] deterioration but also because they are concerned about their coworker. I recall several [supervisors] talking to me about their employees. They were empathic. They were concerned about the nature of their employees' problems apart from the fact that it inhibited functioning. The motive was altruistic.

Indeed, one supervisor expressed her concern for the employee as a person and the pride of being able to reach out to the employee through the EHP.

> I had a young lady [whom] I used to supervise downstairs. I sent her to the psychiatrist. She was a lost case. They [management] wanted me to fire her, and I would not. She has got a family problem; her husband pushes her around. It was a lot of things. I sent her down to Dr. Rose. . . . She is now a happy working girl. A different person! Happily married! So I have done some wonderful things with her.

Employees spoke glowingly of their experiences with the program and its staff. While they appreciate that the program is free of charge and that it is convenient, they are most appreciative of the staff's attitude toward them. Terri A. felt that "it [visiting the EHP] is like sitting and talking to a good friend." Ellen S. agreed: "As far as like talking to someone . . . . I have my whole family and my friends. And, of course, I have got [the therapist]. What other better person could I have than her?" Employees like Deborah F. gave the staff high marks for their professionalism: "It is great, and I have a lot of positive feelings about it. The people I have seen here are very supportive, aware people. I think it is done very professionally." Even when employees' problems were unresolved, they praised the program. Maureen Mc. reported, "I still have problems. At least, I know where they are from. If that is the only thing this place has done for me, then it is great in itself. . . . They [the EHP staff] help a lot."

The EHP's use of medical diagnoses and treatment for family and work problems is a corporate manifestation of medicalization. This medicalization of employee problems is part of a larger phenomenon, the depoliticization of social problems. This is a process that seeks the causes and solutions to complex problems in the individual rather than in the social system (Conrad and Schneider 1980a). It leads to social policies that seek to change the individual rather than the society. In Corpco's EHP, such treatment encourages employees' naïve individualism and discourages them from seeing their problems as class issues. The employees appear to accept the ideology of the Horatio Alger stories and to reject or be oblivious to the notion that social structures affect their opportunities to grow up healthy and to receive good medical care, a decent job, and an adequate income.

The tendency to see the world in individualistic terms was succinctly expressed by Lorraine P., who attributed her sleeplessness and back pain to her blocked promotion and to the conflicts with her new boss. When I asked if she believed her promotion was in jeopardy because of sex discrimination, she replied,

> I do not think it [sex discrimination] is in the company as a whole, but I know for a fact other women . . . [who] worked for this man feel without question that he is one of the . . . unconverted male chauvinists of the company. He is just bad news for any woman who works for him. So, I do not say it is true of the company as a whole. . . . He is noted for it, and I think I was the last to see it because I was brought up that you never cry that any-

thing is unfair, that the world is unfair. It was equally
unfair to everybody, and if you are not succeeding, it is
your own fault. You take that responsibility, and you do
not make excuses.

Although Lorraine could admit that her boss as an individual
was sexually biased, she could not admit that Corpco, as an
organization, might be biased. This is not surprising. Her discussions with her family, network members, Corpco physicians, and the EHP staff encouraged her to think about her
problems in individual terms. All suggested that she get a
transfer, and the EHP recommended biofeedback for her sleeplessness and backaches and pursued its alternative employment strategy with her. By the time I spoke with her, she was
hoping for a transfer and had decided to resign from Corpco
if it did not materialize.

> I have worried about many things most of which never
> happened. I talked about it at home, and we decided that
> if this happens [no transfer], it just is not worth it. Re-
> sign! I have a roof over my head; I have three meals a
> day for the rest of my life, for that matter. You do not
> like to feel that your career has failed. You can get an-
> other job. Maybe you do not get another career. [Another
> job] may never be as well-paying. But [staying] is not
> worth the stress, the blow to pride, and the daily battle
> of wills that is going to occur if I stay here.

Depoliticization during emotional health program treatment aligns well with the individualistic ethic of American
culture. Americans in general are not politically active (Schur
1980), and employees in this sample expressed few if any
political sentiments. The vast majority belonged to nonpo-
litical voluntary organizations (PTA, church groups, athletic
teams) and consider voting the extent of their political activity. Also, they appeared to reject political solutions even when
those solutions are offered. Lorraine P.'s firm rebuff of a woman
activist who tried to persuade her that the decision to resign

was unproductive and a blow to the women's movement is a case in point.

> [The vice president's] assistant came down [to talk with me]. . . . Actually, it was too soon, and it was the wrong approach. She came down and tried to raise hell. She really did not understand things. [She said] I was setting the women's movement back. If I were not a lady, I would have told her what to do with the women's movement. That was the last thing in the world. I could not have cared less. . . . That is not my problem. I thought, "[If] the men didn't understand, that was too damn bad!"

Treatment's tendencies to depoliticize were most clearly expressed by the one employee who had an activist career. Gloria B. came of age in the 1960s, taught in Berkeley, belonged to the National Organization of Women, and developed alternative health care facilities for women in the early 1970s. She originally came to the EHP two years earlier after being divorced by her husband because he disagreed with her activism and losing a custody battle for her two children. She was using the EHP's biofeedback program to learn to cope with stress more effectively. When I asked what two years of therapy and the current biofeedback had given her, Gloria responded,

> . . . confidence in myself. See, I cannot say that before I went to [the therapist]. . . . Nothing that I had ever done in the past made any sense. I made no sense. My value system made no sense. The American judicial system made no sense. . . . It has given me to accept—just to accept. I mean, some of it [the system] is just so outrageous. There is a lot of impotent anger, and I just have to accept it. I guess that is growing up. . . . It is hard. I still want to carry the white flag. The sixties are still there whether I was in the sixties or near the sixties. So we are still fighting all the time. . . . I was in Berkeley. . . I was not a militant. . . I was teaching at the time [and]

163

enough of it was around me that I heard what they believed in. I guess I believed in it too. . . . [Now I realize]
the system is the way the system is. You can manipulate
it a little bit, but it ain't gonna change.

Implications for the future

The EHP solves problems for both management and employees, and its solutions are based upon its own definitions of
the particular problems that employees bring to the program.
These problems are framed within the rationale of cognitive-
behavioral therapy, and EHP solutions are designed to teach
employees to take responsibility for their own problems. Such
treatment helps employees to cope with their problems more
effectively, demonstrates management's humane concerns,
and depoliticizes work problems. To the extent that employees believe that the EHP helps them to overcome their problems, they recognize the EHP's medical expertise, granting it
increased prestige. Likewise, to the extent that managers believe that the EHP helps them to control employees, management recognizes the EHP's medical expertise, granting it
increased prestige.

Several factors, however, moderate the prestige given to the
EHP. First, people do ignore medical advice with which they
do not agree. The vast literature on noncompliance with medical treatment illustrates this point (e.g., Hayes-Bautista 1976;
Sackett and Haynes 1976; Svarstad 1976). Second, the value
of medical expertise may be moderated by the perception of
its cost (Conrad and Schneider 1980a). To be sure, no one is
suggesting that Corpco's EHP program be abandoned, but within
the logic of business, the EHP must weight its financial cost
against its financial benefits to the company so that the greatest cost-effectiveness can be realized.

Historically, management's humanitarian expressions have
been couched in cost-benefit terms. Occupational program
consultants stress that emotional health programs make good
business sense. In the last few years, a small number of cost-

benefit studies on emotional health programs have been completed (e.g., Archer 1977; Foote et al. 1978; Manley et al. 1979; Mannello and Seaman 1979; Schramm et al. 1978). All report significant gains in savings and productivity.

When Corpco's former EHP director evaluated their stress-management training program, he concluded that "cumulative cost-benefit ratios demonstrate that, for every dollar invested in such a program, there is a $5.25 return on that investment." Unfortunately, all these cost-benefit studies suffer from methodological problems and faulty financial assumptions. The Executive Caravan Surveys (Roman 1982; see also Trice and Beyer 1984a) suggest that managers in companies that adopt emotional health programs accept uncritically such cost-benefit arguments. The Executive Caravan Surveys suggest also that, between 1972 and 1979, managers in companies without programs grew increasingly resistant to the belief that emotional health programs are cost effective. This split may mean that program adoption is based partially upon an uncritical acceptance of the belief that humanitarian projects increase productivity; flattering cost-benefit analyses appear to result from efforts to support that ideology and to ensure management's continued financial backing of the programs.

Even though one cannot assert with certainty that emotional health programs are or are not cost effective, what can be asserted is that emotional health programs are becoming big business. Recognition of the EHP's medical expertise is increased by its ability to turn its skills into marketable commodities that can be sold to Corpco's corporate customers. Indeed, this strategy helps to balance the cost-benefit ratio in the EHP's favor, as the current director remarked about the potential profit to Corpco of convincing its corporate clients' employees to stop smoking.

> [The medical director's] primary mandate from the corporation [is] to show a black bottom line. . . . Ultimately, to generate higher income. [For example,] smoke ces-

> sation has been shown to generate a higher income because they [Corpco] have less disability to pay for, and they get longer premiums than expected before they pay out. If it is a 1% change in a $5 billion business, which it was this year, that is a big nut. So that is an expensive thing to look for.

The EHP is developing a smoking-cessation program for Corpco employees and hopes to sell it to corporate clients in the future.

The former director's promotion to vice president of planning and development also suggests Corpco's commitment to marketing the EHP's medical expertise for profit.

> We are getting more into planning and development, and one area . . . is health-system cost containment. I think that [emotional health] programs . . . can be very beneficial at keeping health systems' costs down. . . . So what we are doing is beginning to conceptualize how might we meet the needs of group clients, who come to us saying, "Help us contain health costs."

While the program helps management to demonstrate humane concerns in a cost-effective manner and employees to recontain their problems, these benefits are bought at the expense of the darker consequences, which go to the heart of what it means to be a participant in the workplace. The EHP staff turn all employee problems into medical ones, which require individuals to comply with expert recommendations and assume full responsibility for their concerns. Such compliance and acceptance of responsibility effectively undercuts all group solutions to work-related problems and obscures the meaning of employee behavior within the context of the work system. For example, labeling Salvatore I.'s drinking behavior as alcoholism obscures the fact that his inebriation may be a protest against a demeaning and degrading work situation, and his refusal to comply with the doctor's definition of the problem and his subsequent identity as a malingerer make it easier for Corpco to fire him.

An alternative to rushing employees to treatment is to develop programs that emphasize a balance between constructive confrontation and self-referral. Such a balance would help to protect employees from the darker consequences of medicalization while encouraging the brighter ones. Constructive confrontation, because it is based on the disciplinary process, ensures that employees are sanctioned progressively for unsatisfactory job performance and that, when disputes over sanctions arise, independent arbitrators give employees a fair hearing. In Salvatore's case, this would have meant that his supervisor would have been trained to confront him effectively about his work and that he could have taken his complaints about his supervisor and work situation to arbitration, where the trouble could have been resolved fairly and equitably. Additionally, the progressive sanctions might have motivated him to stop his problem drinking or encouraged him to seek treatment. In contrast to Salvatore, employees such as Terri A., Jeannette T., and Ruth B. appear to have benefited from the opportunity to voluntarily seek help from the emotional health program. A balanced emphasis on self-referral would ensure that services are available to those employees who come to see their troubles as medical problems and that managers are able to express the human side of enterprise.

References

Aday, L.
    1975. Economic and non-economic barriers to the use of needed medical services. *Medical care* 13:447–56.

Alonzo, A.
    1979. Everyday illness behavior: A situational approach to health status deviations. *Social science and medicine* 13A:397–404.

Anderson, V. V.
    1944. Psychiatry in industry. *American journal of psychiatry* 100:134–38.

Archer, J.
    1977. Social stability, work force behavior, and job satisfaction of alcoholic and non-alcoholic blue-collar workers. In *Alcoholism and its treatment in industry*, edited by C. J. Schramm. Baltimore: Johns Hopkins University Press.

Bacon, S.
    1951. Alcoholism and industry. *Civitan magazine* (March): 3–7.
    1948. Alcoholism in industry. *Industrial medicine* 17:161–67.

Bandura, A.
    1977. *Social learning theory.* Englewood Cliffs, N.J.: Prentice-Hall.
    1969. *Principles of behavior modification.* New York: Holt, Rinehart, and Winston.

Beck, A.
    1976. *Cognitive therapy and the emotional disorders.* New York: International University Press.

Becker, H. S.

1973. *Outsiders.* New York: Free Press.

Becker, M.

1979. Psychosocial aspects of health-related behavior. In *Handbook of medical sociology,* 3d ed., edited by H. Freeman et al. Englewood Cliffs, N.J.: Prentice-Hall.

Belasco, J. A., and Trice, H. M.

1969. *The assessment of change in training and therapy.* New York: McGraw-Hill.

Benson, H.

1975. *The relaxation response.* New York: Morrow.

Beyer, J., et al.

1980. The impact of federal sector unions on supervisors' use of personnel policies. *Industrial and labor relations review* 33:212–31.

Blum, J. D.

1980. Compensating the mentally impaired worker. In *Mental wellness programs for employees,* edited by R. H. Egdahl and D. C. Walsh. New York: Springer-Verlag.

Boyer, R. O., and Morais, H. M.

1970. *Labor's untold story.* New York: United Electrical, Radio, and Machine Workers of America.

Brandes, S. D.

1970. *American welfare capitalism.* Chicago: University of Chicago Press.

Braverman, H.

1974. *Labor and monopoly capital.* New York: Monthly Review Press.

Brockman, J., et al.

1979. Facts or artifacts? Changing public attitudes toward the mentally ill. *Social science and medicine* 13A:673–82.

Brown, B. B.

1980. *Supermind: The ultimate energy.* New York: Harper and Row.

Brunswick, A., et al.

1979. Who sees the doctor? A study of urban black adolescents. *Social science and medicine* 13A:45–56.

Bullough, V. L.

1976. *Sexual variance in society and history.* New York: John Wiley and Sons.

Burling, T., and Longaker, W.
    1955. Training for industrial psychiatry. *American journal of psychiatry* 111:493.
Burlingame, C. C.
    1946. Psychiatry in industry. *American journal of psychiatry* 103:549–53.
Byers, B.
    1979. ALMACA's national EAP survey is summarized. *The ALMACAN* 9 (November):1–2.
Campbell, C. M.
    1943. The psychiatrist and industrial organization. *Journal of psychiatry* 100:286–87.
Carey, A.
    1967. The Hawthorne studies: A radical criticism. *American sociological review* 32:403–17.
Carneiro, R. L., ed.
    1967. *The evolution of society: Selections from Herbert Spencer's* Principles of Sociology. Chicago: University of Chicago Press.
Carter, I.
    1977. Social work in industry: A history and a viewpoint. *Social thought* 3 (Winter):7–31.
Cohen, W. J.
    1973. Revolution in mental health. In *Industrial mental health and employee counseling*, edited by R. L. Nolan. New York: Behavioral Publications.
Conrad, P.
    1976. *Identifying hyperactive children: The medicalization of deviant behavior*. Lexington, Mass.: D. C. Heath.
Conrad, P., and Schneider, J.
    1980a. *Deviance and medicalization: From badness to sickness*. St. Louis: C. V. Mosby Co.
    1980b. Looking at levels of medicalization: A comment on Strong's critique of the thesis of medical imperialism. *Social science and medicine* 14A:75–79.
Coser, L.
    1964. *Functions of social conflict*. New York: Free Press.
Daniels, A. K.
    1972. Military psychiatry: The emergence of a subspecialty. In *Medical men and their work*, edited by E. Freidson

171

and J. Lorber. Chicago: Aldine.

1969. The captive professional: Bureaucratic limitations in the practice of military psychiatry. *Journal of health and social behavior* 10:255–65.

Davidson, P. O., and Davidson, S. M., eds.

1980. *Behavioral medicine: Changing health lifestyles.* New York: Brunner/Mazel.

Davis, K.

1938. Mental hygiene and social structure. *Psychiatry* 1:55–65.

Denenberg, T. S., and Denenberg, R. V.

1983. *Alcohol and drugs: Issues in the workplace.* Washington, D.C.: Bureau of National Affairs.

Denzin, N. K.

1978. *The research act.* Chicago: Aldine.

Dershimer, F. W.

1955. Psychiatry in industry. *American journal of psychiatry* 111:534–35.

1954. Psychiatry in industry. *American journal of psychiatry* 110:527–28.

1953. Psychiatry in industry. *American journal of psychiatry* 109:524–26.

1952. Psychiatry in industry. *American journal of psychiatry* 108:536–38.

Diamond, T.

1983. Nursing homes as trouble. *Urban life* 12, 3:269–86.

Dickson, W., and Roethlisberger, F. J.

1966. *Counseling in an organization.* Cambridge, Mass.: Harvard University Press.

Drucker, P.

1974. *Management: Tasks, responsibilities, and practices.* New York: Harper and Row.

Dunkin, W. S.

1982. *The EAP manual.* New York: National Council on Alcoholism.

Edwards, R.

1979. *Contested terrain: The transformation of the workplace in the twentieth century.* New York: Basic Books.

Eilbert, H.

1959. The development of personnel management in the United States. *Business history review* 33:345–64.

Ellis, A., and Grieger, R., eds.
   1977. *Handbook of rational-emotive therapy.* New York: Springer.
Emerson, R. M., and Messinger, S. L.
   1977. The micro-politics of trouble. *Social problems* 25:121–34.
Erikson, K. T.
   1966. *Wayward puritans.* New York: John Wiley and Sons.
Fabrega, H.
   1973. Toward a model of illness behavior. *Medical care* 11:470–84.
Ferguson, C. A., and Fersing, J. E.
   1965. *The legacy of neglect.* Fort Worth, Texas: Industrial Mental Health Associates.
Ferraro, K. J.
   1983. Negotiating trouble in a battered women's shelter. *Urban life* 12, 3:287–306.
Filstead, W. J.
   1979. Qualitative methods: A needed perspective in evaluation research. In *Qualitative and quantitative methods in evaluation research*, edited by T. D. Cook and C. S. Reichardt. Beverly Hills, Calif.: Sage Publications.
Filstead, W. J., ed.
   1970. *Qualitative methodology: Firsthand involvement with the social world.* Chicago: Markham Publishing Company.
Foote, A., et al.
   1978. *Cost effectiveness of occupational employee assistance programs.* Ann Arbor, Mich.: University of Michigan.
Fox, R.
   1957. Training for uncertainty. In *The student physician*, edited by R. K. Merton et al. Cambridge, Mass.: Harvard University Press.
Freedburg, E. J., and Johnston, W. E.
   1979. Changes in drinking behavior, employment status, and other life areas for employed alcoholics after treatment. *Journal of drug issues* 9:523–34.
Freidlander, F., and Brown, L. D.
   1974. Organizational development. *Annual review of psychology* 25:313–41.

Freidson, E.

  1970. *Profession of medicine.* New York: Harper and Row.

  1961. *Patients' views of medical practice.* New York: Russell Sage Foundation.

Fries, B. E., and Ginsberg, A. S.

  1979. The effect of delay rules in controlling unscheduled visits to hospitals. *Medical care* 17:967–72.

Geertz, C.

  1973. *The interpretation of cultures.* New York: Basic Books.

Geiser, R. L.

  1976. *Behavior mod and the managed society.* Boston: Beacon Press.

Giberson, L. G.

  1936. Psychiatry in industry. *Personnel journal* 15:91–95.

Glaser, B., and Strauss, A.

  1967. *The discovery of grounded theory.* Chicago: Aldine.

Glasser, M., et al.

  1975. Obstacles to utilization of prepaid mental health care. *American journal of psychiatry* 132:710–15.

Goffman, E.

  1963. *Stigma.* Englewood Cliffs, N.J.: Prentice-Hall.

  1961. *Asylums.* Garden City, N.Y.: Doubleday and Company.

Goldbeck, W.

  1979. Employee mental wellness programs and issues: An overview. Paper prepared by the Washington Business Group on Health.

Googins, B., and Kurtz, N. R.

  1981. Discriminating supervisors in occupational programs. *Journal of drug issues* 11, 2:199–216.

  1979. Supervisory networks: Toward an alternative training model. *Labor-management alcoholism journal* (July–August).

Gordon, G.

  1973. Industrial psychiatry—Five year plant experience. In *Industrial mental health and employee counseling,* edited by R. L. Nolan. New York: Behavioral Publications.

Greenley, J. R., and Mechanic, D.

  1976. Social selection in seeking help for psychological problems. *Journal of health and social behavior* 17:249–62.

Halleck, S. L.
1972. *The politics of therapy.* New York: Harper and Row.
Hawkins, R., and Tiedeman, G.
1975. *The creation of deviance: Interpersonal and organizational determinants.* Columbus, Ohio: Bell and Howell Company.
Hayes-Bautista, D. E.
1976. Modifying the treatment: Patient compliance, patient control, and medical care. *Social science and medicine* 10:233–38.
Hellan, R.
1981. National Employee Assistance Providers Association information letter dated August 14.
Henderson, R., and Bacon, S.
1953. Problem drinking: The Yale Plan for Business and Industry. *Quarterly journal of studies on alcohol* 14:247–62.
Heyman, M.
1978. *Alcoholism programs in industry.* New Brunswick, N.J.: Rutgers Center of Alcohol Studies.
1976. Referral to alcoholism programs in industry: Coercion, confrontation, and choice. *Journal of studies on alcohol* 37:900–907.
Holmes, T. H., and Rahe, R. H.
1967. The social readjustment rating scale. *Journal of psychosomatic research* 11:213–18.
Horwitz, A.
1977. The pathways into psychiatric treatment: Some differences between men and women. *Journal of health and social behavior* 18:169–78.
Hughes, E. C.
1962. Good people and dirty work. *Social problems* 10:3–11.
Jacobson, A. M., et al.
1978. Factors relating to the use of mental health services in a neighborhood health care center. *Public health reports* 93:232–39.
Jellinek, E. M.
1947. What shall we do about alcoholism? *Vital speeches* 13:252–54.

Jenkins, D.
> 1973. *Job power: Blue and white collar democracy.* New York: Penguin Books.

Kadushin, C.
> 1969. *Why people go to psychiatrists.* New York: Atherton Press.
> 1967. Social class and ill health: The need for further research. *Sociological inquiry* 37:323–32.

Kahne, M. J., and Schwartz, C. G.
> 1978. Negotiating trouble: The social construction and management of trouble in a college psychiatric context. *Social problems* 25:461–75.

Kanter, R. M.
> 1977. *Men and women of the corporation.* New York: Basic Books.

Kiefhaber, A., and Goldbeck, W. B.
> 1979. A WBGH survey on employee mental wellness programs. Mimeographed. Washington Business Group on Health.

Kosa, J., and Robertson, L. S.
> 1969. The social aspects of health and illness. In *Poverty and health,* edited by J. Kosa et al. Cambridge, Mass.: Harvard University Press.

Kulka, R. A., et al.
> 1979. Social class and the use of professional help for personal problems: 1957–1976. *Journal of health and social behavior* 20:2–17.

Kurtz, N. R., et al.
> 1980. Supervisors' views of an occupational alcoholism program: An experiential perspective. *Alcohol, health and research world* (Spring).

Laing, R. D.
> 1965. *The divided self.* Baltimore: Penguin Books.

Lawler, E. E.
> 1976. Control systems in organizations. In *Handbook of industrial and organizational psychology,* edited by M. Dunnette. Chicago: Rand-McNally.

Likert, R.
> 1967. *The human organization: Its management and value.* New York: McGraw-Hill.

Lott, G. M.
  1946. Emotional first-aid stations in industry. *Industrial medicine* 15:419–22.

Lublin, J. S.
  1980. On-the-job stress leads many workers to file—and win —compensation awards. *Wall Street journal*, September 17:33.

Luft, H. S., et al.
  1976. Factors affecting the use of physician services in a rural community. *American journal of public health* 66:865–71.

McGregor, D. M.
  1960. *The human side of enterprise.* New York: McGraw-Hill.

McKinlay, J.
  1972. Some approaches and problems in the study of the use of services: An overview. *Journal of health and social behavior* 13:115–52.

McLean, A.
  1973. Occupational mental health: Review of an emerging art. In *Industrial mental health and employee counseling,* edited by R. L. Noland. New York: Behavioral Publications.

Manley, T., et al.
  1979. Alcoholism and alcohol related problems among USAF civilian employees. *AFIT technical report,* 79-4 US Air Force. Fairborn, Ohio: Air Force University.

Mannello, T. A., and Seaman, F. J.
  1979. Prevalence, costs, and handling of drinking problems on seven railroads: Final report. Mimeographed. Washington, D.C.: University Research Corporation.

Mannheim, K.
  1936. *Ideology and utopia.* New York: Harcourt Brace and Company.

Mayo, E.
  1923. Irrationality and reverie. *Journal of personnel research* 1:477–83.

Mechanic, D.
  1968. *Medical sociology: A selective view.* New York: Free Press.

Meichenbaum, D.
    1977. *Cognitive behavior modification.* New York: Plenum Press.

Mumm, E. W., and Spiegel, W. R.
    1962. *Mental health in industry.* Personnel Study No. 15. Bureau of Business Research, University of Texas.

Nelson, D., and Campbell, S.
    1972. Taylorism versus welfare work in American industry, H. L. Gantt and the Bancrofts. *Business history review* 46:1–16.

Noble, D. F.
    1977. *America by design: Science, technology, and the rise of corporate capitalism.* Oxford: Oxford University Press.

Noland, R. L., ed.
    1973. *Industrial mental health and employee counseling.* New York: Behavioral Publications.

Opinion Research Corporation.
    1966. Mental health in the corporation. *Public opinion index for industry* 24, 5.

O'Toole, J.
    1973. *Work in America.* Cambridge, Mass.: MIT Press.

O'Toole, P.
    1980. The menace of the corporate shrink. *Savvy* (October): 49–52.

Ouchi, W., and Jaeger, A.
    1978. Social structure and organizational type. In *Environment and organizations,* edited by M. Meyer et al. San Francisco: Jossey-Bass.

Parsons, T.
    1951. *The social system.* New York: Free Press.

Patton, M. Q.
    1980. *Qualitative evaluation methods.* Beverly Hills, Calif.: Sage Publications.

Peel, J. D. Y., ed.
    1982. *Herbert Spencer on social evolution: Selected writings.* Chicago: University of Chicago Press.

Perlis, L.
    1980. Labor and employee assistance programs. In *Mental wellness programs for employees,* edited by R. H. Egdahl and D. C. Walsh. New York: Springer-Verlag.

Perrow, C.
    1972. *Complex organizations: A critical essay.* Glenview, Ill.: Scott, Foresman and Company.
Peyrot, M.
    1985. Coerced voluntarism: The micro-politics of drug treatment. *Urban life* 13, 4:343–65.
Phillips, D.
    1963. Rejection: A possible consequence of seeking help for mental disorders. *American sociological review* 28:963–72.
Presnall, L. F.
    1966. Alcoholism and employees. Paper presented at the University of Utah School of Alcohol Studies, June 14.
    1956. People, production, and personnel counseling. Paper presented to the New Mexico Mining Association Convention, Carlsbad, New Mexico, November 1.
Reynolds, B. C.
    1975. *Social work and social living.* NASW classics. Washington, D. C.: NASW.
Ritzer, G., and Trice, H. M.
    1969. *An occupation in conflict.* Ithaca, N.Y.: New York State School of Industrial and Labor Relations.
Roethlisberger, F. J., and Dickson, W. J.
    1939. *Management and the worker.* Cambridge, Mass.: Harvard University Press.
Roman, P. M.
    1982. Employee alcoholism programs in major corporations in 1979: Scope, change, and receptivity. *Prevention, intervention, and treatment: Concerns and models.* Alcohol and health monograph no. 3. Rockville, Md.: U.S. Dept. of Health and Human Services.
    1981a. From employee alcoholism to employee assistance: Deemphases on prevention and alcohol problems in work-based programs. *Journal of studies on alcohol* 42:244–72.
    1981b. Job characteristics and the identification of deviant drinking. *Journal of drug issues* 11, 3:357–64.
    1980. Medicalization and social control in the workplace: Prospects for the 1980s. *Journal of applied behavioral sciences* 16:407–22.

Roman, P. M., and Trice, H. M.
  1976. Alcohol abuse and work organizations. In *The biology of alcoholism.* Vol. 4, edited by B. Kissin and H. Begleiter. New York: Plenum Press.

Rosenbaum, M., and Romano, J.
  1943. Psychiatric casualties among defense workers. *American journal of psychiatry* 100:314–19.

Rosenhan, D. L.
  1973. On being sane in insane places. *Science* 179:250–58.

Rosenstock, I. M.
  1966. Why people use health services. *Millbank Memorial Fund quarterly* (pt. 2) 44:94–127.

Sackett, D. L., and Haynes, B. R.
  1976. *Compliance with therapeutic regimens.* Baltimore: Johns Hopkins University Press.

Scheff, T. J.
  1968. Negotiating reality: Notes on power in the assessment of responsibility. *Social problems* 16:3–17.
  1966. *Being mentally ill.* Chicago: Aldine.

Schneider, J., and Conrad, P.
  1980. In the closet with illness: Epilepsy, stigma potential and information control. *Social problems* 28:32–44.

Schrag, P.
  1978. *Mind control.* New York: Delta Books.

Schramm, C., et al.
  1978. *Workers who drink: Their treatment in an industrial setting.* Lexington, Mass.: D. C. Heath.

Schur, E. M.
  1980. *The politics of deviance: Stigma contests and the uses of power.* Englewood Cliffs, N.J.: Prentice-Hall.
  1979. *Interpreting deviance.* New York: Harper and Row.
  1971. *Labeling deviant behavior.* New York: Harper and Row.

Schwartz, C. G., and Kahne, M. J.
  1983. Medical help as negotiated achievement. *Psychiatry* 46:333–50.
  1977. The social construction of trouble and its implications for psychiatrists working in college settings. *Journal of the American College Health Association* 25:194–97.

Scott, W. G., and Hart, D. K.
  1979. *Organizational America.* Boston: Houghton Mifflin.

References

Shaffir, W. B., et al., eds.

1980. *Fieldwork experience: Qualitative approaches to social research.* New York: St. Martin's Press.

Shain, M., and Walden, P.

1980. Employee assistance programs as conflict-avoiding devices and the influence of arbitral decisions on their development. In *Employee assistance programs: Philosophy, theory, and practice,* edited by M. Shain and J. Groeneveld. Lexington, Mass.: Lexington Books.

Christopher D. Smithers Foundation.

1958. *A basic outline for a company program.*

Sobel, D.

1981. Thousands with mental health insurance choose to pay own bill. *New York times,* August 4:C1–2.

Southard, E. E.

1920. The modern specialist in unrest: A place for the psychiatrist in industry. *Mental hygiene* 4:550.

Spitzer, S.

1975. Toward a marxian theory of deviance. *Social problems* 22:638–51.

Spradley, J. P.

1979. *The ethnographic interview.* New York: Holt, Rinehart, and Winston.

Strauss, G.

1969. Human relations, 1968 style. *Industrial relations* 7, 3:262–76.

Suchman, E.

1966. Health orientation and medical care. *Journal of public health* 56:97–105.

1965. Stages of illness and medical care. *Journal of health and human behavior* 6:114–28.

1964. Sociomedical variations among ethnic groups. *American journal of sociology* 70:319–331.

Sudnow, D.

1965. Normal crimes: Sociological features of the penal code. *Social problems* 12:255–71.

Svarstad, B.

1976. Physician-patient communication and patient conformity with medical advice. In *The growth of bureaucratic medicine,* edited by D. Mechanic. New York: John Wiley

181

and Sons.

Sykes, A. J. M.

1965. Economic interest and the Hawthorne researchers. *Human relations* 18:253–63.

Szasz, T. S.

1970. *Ideology and insanity.* Garden City, N.Y.: Doubleday and Company.

1961. *The myth of mental illness.* New York: Paul B. Hoeber.

Taylor, F. W.

1911. *The principles of scientific management.* New York: Harper and Row.

Telles, J. L., and Pollack, M. H.

1981. Feeling sick: The experience and legitimation of illness. *Social science and medicine* 15A:243–51.

Trice, H. M., and Beyer, J. M.

1984a. Employee assistance programs: Blending performance-oriented and humanitarian ideologies to assist emotionally disturbed employees. In *Research in community and mental health.* Vol. 4, edited by J. R. Greenley. Greenwich, Conn.: JAI Press.

1984b. Work-related outcomes of constructive confrontation strategies in a job-based alcoholism program. *Journal of studies on alcohol* 45, 5:393–404.

1981a. A data-based examination of selection bias in the evaluation of a job-based alcoholism program. *Alcoholism: Clinical and experimental research* 5, 4:489–96.

1981b. Job-based alcoholism programs: Motivating problem-drinkers to rehabilitation. In *American handbook of alcoholism,* edited by E. M. Pattison and E. Kaufmann. New York: Gardner Press.

Trice, H. M., et al.

1981. Sowing seeds of change: How work organizations in New York State responded to occupational program consultants. *Journal of drug issues* 11:311–36.

Trice, H. M., and Roman, P. M.

1978. *Spirits and demons at work: Alcohol and other drugs on the job.* 2d ed. Ithaca, N.Y.: New York State School of Industrial and Labor Relations, Cornell University.

Trice, H. M., and Schonbrunn, M.
   1981. A history of job-based alcoholism programs: 1900–1955. *Journal of drug issues* 11:171–98.
Turner, R. J.
   1981. Social support as a contingency in psychological well-being. *Journal of health and social behavior* 22:357–67.
Vanek, J.
   1975. *Self-management: Economic liberation of man.* Middlesex, England: Penguin Books.
Veroff, J., et al.
   1981. *Mental health in America: Patterns of help-seeking from 1957 to 1976.* New York: Basic Books.
Vonachen, H. A., et al.
   1946. A comprehensive mental hygiene program at Caterpillar Tractor Co. *Industrial medicine* 15:179–84.
Von Wiegand, R.
   1971. The problem of alcoholism. *Environmental control and safety management.* Reprint (March).
Weinberg, M. S.
   1978. The nudist management of respectability. In *Deviance: The interactionist perspective*, edited by E. Rubington and M. S. Weinberg. New York: Macmillan Publishing Company.
Weiss, R.
   1980. *Dealing with alcoholism in the workplace.* New York: Conference Board.
Whyte, W. F.
   1984. *Learning from the field.* Beverly Hills, Calif.: Sage Publications.
   1979. On making the most of participant observation. *American sociologist* 14 (February):56–66.
Whyte, W. F., et al.
   1983. *Worker participation and ownership: Cooperative strategies for strengthening local economies.* Ithaca, N.Y.: ILR Press.
Whyte, W. H.
   1957. *The organization man.* New York: Doubleday Anchor Books.

183

Wiener, C. L.

    1981. *The politics of alcoholism: Building an arena around a social problem.* New Brunswick, N.J.: Transaction Books.

Williams, A. W., et al.

    1981. A model of mental health, life events, and social supports applicable to general populations. *Journal of health and social behavior* 22:324–36.

Witti, F.

    1980. The capitol connection. *EAP digest* (November-December):11.

Wrich, J. T.

    1980. *The employee assistance program: Updated for the 1980s.* Center City, Minn.: Hazelden.

    1974. *The employee assistance program.* Center City, Minn.: Hazelden.

Wriston, W. B.

    1980. Address to the Conference on Employee Mental Wellness. In *Mental wellness programs for employees,* edited by R. H. Egdahl and D. C. Walsh. New York: Springer-Verlag.

Yarrow, M., et al.

    1955. The psychological meaning of mental illness in the family. *Journal of social issues* 11:12–24.

Zola, I. K.

    1973. Pathways to the doctor—From person to patient. *Social science and medicine* 7:677–89.

    1972. Studying the decision to see a doctor. *Advances in psychosomatic medicine* 8:216–36.

    1966. Culture and symptoms: An analysis of presenting complaints. *American sociological review* 31:615–30.

    1964. Illness behavior of the working class: Implications and recommendations. In *Blue collar world: Studies of the American worker,* edited by A. Shostak and W. Gomberg. Englewood Cliffs, N.J.: Prentice-Hall.

Zusman, J.

    1976. *Mental health: N.Y. law and practice.* Matthew Bender.

Zwerdling, D.

    1980. *Democracy at work: A guide to workplace ownership, participation, and self-management experiments in the United States and Europe.* New York: Harper and Row.

Index

DATE DUE